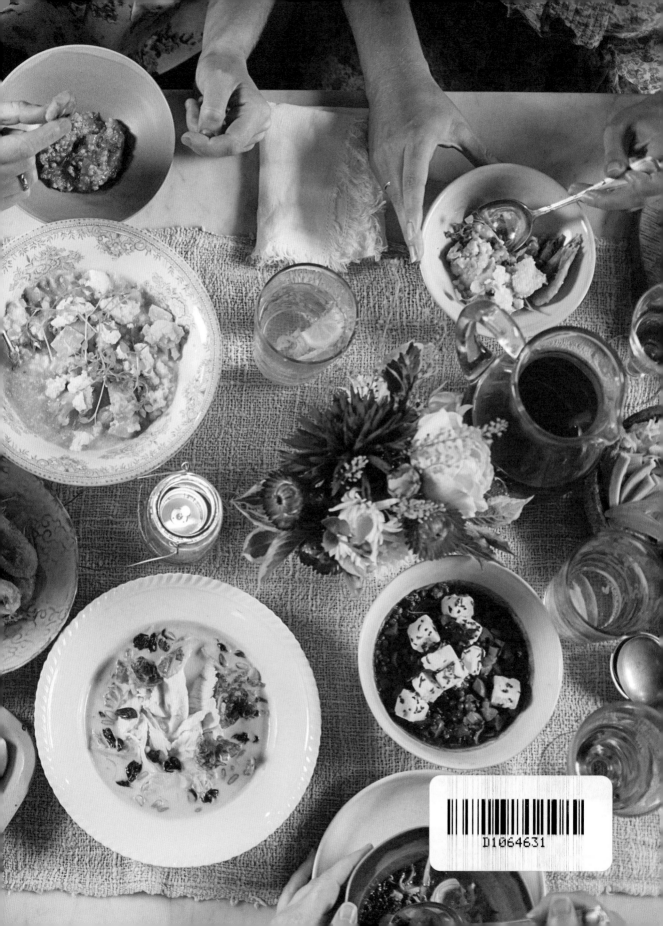

MAGIC SOUP

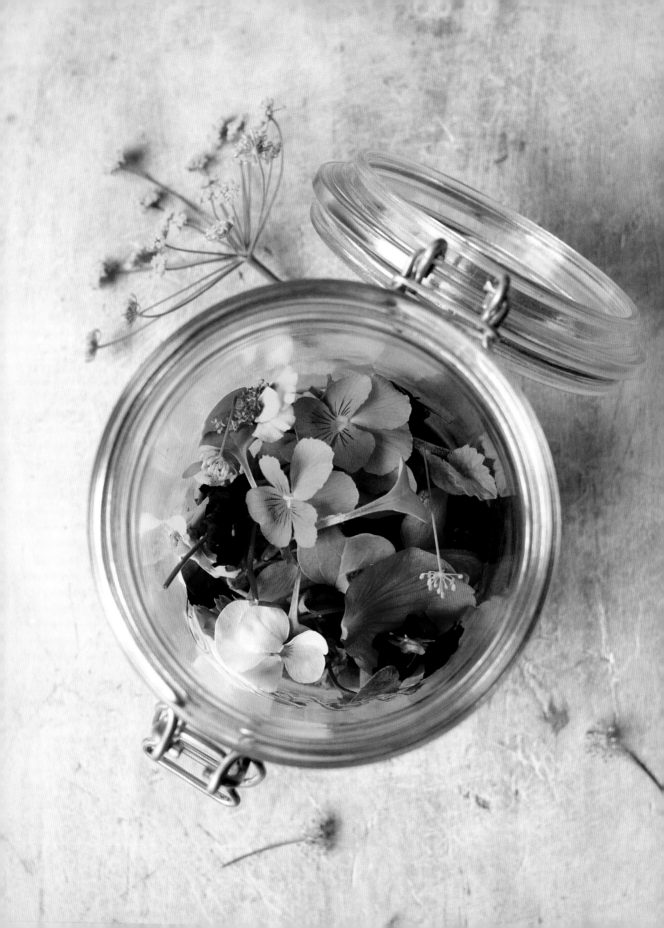

Nicole Pisani and Kate Adams

MAGIC SOUP

FOOD FOR HEALTH AND HAPPINESS

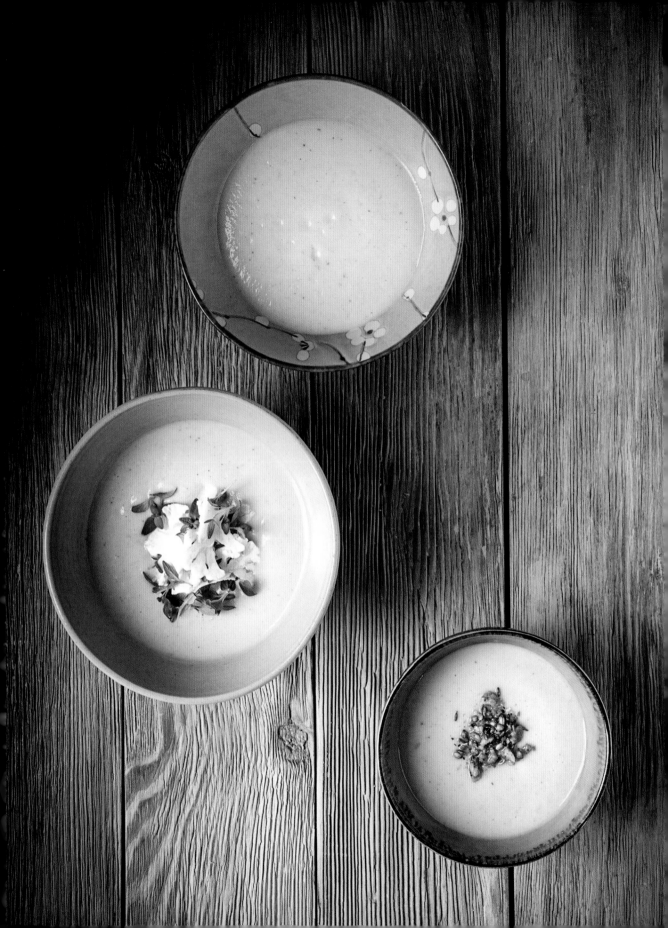

CONTENTS

INTRODUCTION

We are a chef (Nicole) and a writer (Kate), and we love soup. It takes us back to basics, to the essence of simple food for the body and soul. When you eat a really good bowl of soup, it puts you in a positive frame of mind, and you know you're nourishing your body, too. Making soup is like therapy: it's relaxing, creative and generous.

For both of us, eating is emotional, and we think that's a great thing. Food should be a source of passion, of delight. Nicole can tell how a person is feeling the moment she walks into their kitchen: whether they're at one with their world or in need of a 'kitchen cleanse' (in other words, their cupboards are cluttered with lots of delicious ingredients forgotten and left unseen and unused in the corners). We can feel it, too, when we get trapped in unhealthy eating patterns and need to make a new start. For us, the first step is usually making a fresh soup to rekindle our desire for health and happiness.

Our aim is to show that cooking at home is the simple, unscientific but real-life answer to healthy living. When you cook and eat from scratch, there's very little that isn't good for you in moderation; at the very least, every recipe and every meal can have a bit of magic in it. Depending on what we need and what we fancy, soup can be comforting, a quick lunchtime fix or a feast for the gods. As early as humans could build fires and make watertight pots, they made soups and stews with the ingredients they had to hand, and that tradition continues. Nicole will often make 'everything left in the fridge' soup, her own version of hunter-gathering, or an ode to Scotland with the Hotch Potch soup. Chicken soup makes us feel better when we're poorly, while Miso or Kitchari are the perfect start to a healthy cleanse.

Cooking gathers people together, over the stove or at the table. It's generous and giving, and sitting and chatting is as nourishing as the food itself. There is a beautiful Latvian proverb that says 'a smile is half the meal': there are times when cooking is a way to get back to the important things in life, whether you're taking a delicious, healthy lunch to work in a Thermos flask or roasting a few vegetables with herbs or spices and making a simple soup for a busy week ahead.

Close your eyes and imagine everything you need for a good meal. Then make soup!

'SOUP OF THE EVENING, BEAUTIFUL SOUP!'

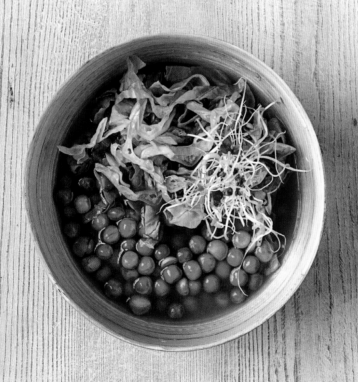

THE MOCK TURTLE IN *ALICE'S ADVENTURES IN WONDERLAND* (1865)

HOW IT ALL BEGAN

'I live on good soup, not on fine words.' MOLIÈRE (1622–1673)

One day, Kate was telling Nicole how making soup had helped her start cooking at home more, as well as improving her health; she found soups fulfilling and delicious, and happened to lose weight at the same time. The first time she made Portuguese Chicken, Lemon and Mint soup she devoured it, wondering how she could have forgotten just how good soup can be. It wasn't a short-term fix either: years later, she still hasn't put the weight back on because she enjoyed the change and it had become a part of her lifestyle.

Nicole, meanwhile, has always been passionate about making people happy through food and inspiring them to cook. After cooking for the homeless and on Zen retreats, she's spent a lot of time thinking about how to get a whole day's nutrition into one bowl of soup. She was also inspired during her time working for Anna Hansen and Yotam Ottolenghi at The Modern Pantry and Nopi restaurants in London. Both Anna and Yotam encouraged their staff to share food, to eat together and cook together. For Nicole, the greatest compliment you can give her is your empty bowl.

When Kate was in Mauritius – an island of amazingly healthy people – she heard about Magic Soup, which was really just a brilliant way to describe a simple vegetable soup that's packed with goodness and spices, which women traditionally ate after having a baby. It would give them lots of nutrition while gently helping them get their figure back, too.

So together we planted the seed of an idea, which eventually grew into *Magic Soup*.

We've had some real adventures while creating the soups in this book. Kate learned how to make soup with a whole chicken, and from having no idea what spice mixes like dukkah or za'atar were, she now cooks with them freely and easily. Nicole never thought she would like herbal tea until she created salmon poached in lemongrass tea. That's the only rule we have: they just need to *taste good*. We're not interested in taking the joy of out food. What makes us happy is that each and every recipe has a little bit of magic in it, whether it will comfort you on a rainy day, make you eat too fast because it's so delicious, or make you feel good about what you ate today. There are healing soups and New Year soups, chilled soups for hot summer days and warm, toasty soups for winter evenings. There are soups to cleanse the body and soothe the soul; some will take you to far off countries, while others will bring you home. We hope it rekindles your love of soup and gives you some ideas to inspire you, so that you'll often be able to say: 'Oh, I know what we'll have tonight…'

A SHORT HISTORY OF SOUP

'The transformation which occurs in the cauldron is quintessential and wondrous, subtle and delicate.' I YIN (239 BC)

Soup came into being about five millennia ago when human beings began to farm and cultivate food in addition to hunting and gathering, and it marked a crucial stage in their development. When people began to put different ingredients in a pot with water over the heat of the fire, they created broths, gruel and stews. Before this, food had always been either roasted, fried or baked separately. The discovery of boiling and simmering meant that a much greater variety of plants and grains could be combined and added to the diet, and meat could provide even more nutrition through boiling the bones.

The word 'soup' most likely derives from the bread over which broth was poured, the 'sup' or 'sop'. The first restaurants, as we now think of them, appeared in Paris in the eighteenth century and served soups, which were usually meat consommés or bouillons that would help to 'restore' a person's strength and vitality, or cure a hangover. Bone-based broths had been used for centuries and across cultures as healing remedies, and chicken soup is worthy of a book of its own.

In the nineteenth century the first packet soups appeared, known as 'pocket soups'. As transportation improved and travel became more possible, portable canned and dehydrated soups grew in popularity. The Campbell's Soup Company opened its first factory in 1869 in Camden, New Jersey, and the first can of tomato soup was produced in 1895. These days, we like soups to taste as fresh as possible, and to offer seasonal specialities and super-healthy ingredients – but sometimes this goes too far. The Cabbage Soup Diet became famous in the 1970s and was notorious for its lack of flavour and variety, and unfortunate side effects. Maybe that's why nobody has ever actually claimed to have invented the diet, despite the millions of people who tried it.

For us, though, soup reminds us of our families, our travels and our discoveries. Kate never thought she'd eat a mung bean until she discovered Kitchari; we had no idea that Peanut Butter Soup could be so good, or how many wonderful and varied soups have overcooked rice in common, from Congee in China to Avgolemono in Spain. From the far corners of the globe to your own back garden, you will find the ingredients for soup. Grab whatever you happen to have in your cupboard today and get chopping!

SOUP ESSENTIALS

EQUIPMENT

Having the right equipment in the kitchen makes life so much easier, but there's a fine line between having what you need and overcrowding your counters with gadgets you'll hardly ever use. One really good knife is a better investment than a whole set, for example. The same is true for pots and pans; Kate's mum splashed out on three Le Creuset pans when she and her sister were tiny, and they still have pride of place in her sister's kitchen decades later.

Blenders
A basic jug blender is incredibly useful, and a handheld stick blender can help to reduce the washing up. There are now specially designed soup-maker blenders available, so that you can sauté your vegetables, then add your stock and blend all in the same appliance: nifty!

Flasks
Wide-brimmed flasks are great for transporting soup. You can also buy microwaveable plastic flasks, so you can transfer your soup straight from the refrigerator to work and heat it up at lunchtime. Thermal bento box sets from Japan are gaining popularity, and these often include a soup flask plus a couple of containers for salads or rice.

Tupperware
As you might expect from a chef, Nicole has a towering collection of Tupperware. Her top tip is to use the size that leaves the least room for air at the top, and that way your soup (or whatever you're storing) will last a bit longer. The vegetable and chicken soups are the easiest to store, and are best eaten within two days if kept in the fridge, or up to a month in the freezer.

STORECUPBOARD

It pays to give your storecupboards a good clean and tidy-up every now and then. That way you can see exactly what you have, rather than leaving lots of wonderful spices or grains unused and going stale where you can't see them. Nicole uses a drawer for spices, rather than a cupboard, because she can see them all and choose the one she fancies. We also try to grow as many fresh herbs as possible and always keep a few pastes and mustards in the fridge.

If you can get to an Asian supermarket, you can stock up without spending a great deal. We pick up bags of frozen kaffir lime leaves and lemongrass as well as generous bottles of fish sauce, rice wine, noodles and soy sauces. For spice blends, the supermarkets are beginning to stock many more varieties, and we also shop online once in a while (see page 82) to replenish our favourites.

Spices

Black onion seeds
Black sesame seeds
Cardamom pods
  (green)
Coriander seeds
Chilli powder
Chinese five-spice
Cinnamon (sticks and
  ground)
Cloves (whole)
Cumin seeds
Fennel seeds
Ginger (ground)
Juniper berries
Mustard seeds
Nigella seeds
Paprika (smoked and
  sweet)
Peppercorns (black
  and pink)
Star anise
Sumac
Turmeric (ground or
  whole if you can
  find it)

Nuts & seeds

Pine nuts
Pumpkin seeds
Sesame seeds

Sauces & pastes

Coconut milk
Fish sauce
Harissa
Mirin
Miso pastes
Sundried tomato
  paste
Sweet chilli sauce
Tamari (wheat-free soy
  sauce)
Tamarind
Tomato purée
Ponzu (citrus soy
  sauce)

Dried herbs
& aromatics

Bay leaves
Curry leaves
Garlic
Ginger
Lemongrass
Mint

Starches

Amaranth
Buckwheat
Farro
Freekeh
Giant couscous
Millet
Noodles (brown rice,
  soba, udon)
Orzo pasta
Pearl barley
Quinoa
Rice (brown, long
  grain, Thai black,
  wild)

Oils & vinegars

Apple cider vinegar
Balsamic vinegar
Coconut oil
Extra-virgin olive oil
Groundnut oil
Light olive oil
Sesame oil
Sherry vinegar
Vegetable/sunflower
  oil

Others

Instant stock powder
  (our favourites are
  Kallo or Marigold)
Panko breadcrumbs
Honey
Mustard (English,
  Dijon and
  wholegrain)

NOTES FOR COOKS

We've included lots of recipes for salads and other garnishes we like to enjoy with our soups. These are always optional, but if you have the time and inclination they are designed to add the perfect balance of flavour or crunch. If you're making a blended vegetable soup, for example, try taking a few moments to toast some nuts or seeds or chop a handful of fresh herbs.

Most of the recipes can be adapted to be dairy and/or gluten free. Swap butter for olive oil or occasionally coconut oil, which is becoming a favourite of ours. We love using nut milks, such as almond, hazelnut and coconut, instead of cows' milk. If we have specified a wheat grain such as farro or couscous in a recipe, you can swap in any gluten-free grain or seed you enjoy, such as quinoa, amaranth or buckwheat. We didn't really know what to do with millet until we started using it in soups, where we have discovered it gives a gentle heartiness.

Using your own homemade stock will always add depth of flavour, so if you have a few spare vegetables, put a pot on the stove for an hour. There are now a lot of good shop-bought stocks available, too, and we will quite happily use vegetable bouillon or meat stocks when we haven't had time to make our own.

We're snobs when it comes to salt, and always use a good-quality flaky sea salt. We aren't snobs when it comes to olive oil for cooking, though, because the lighter varieties are better for cooking at high temperatures; but when finishing a soup we like to push the boat out with a little extra-virgin olive oil, and we love infusing olive oil with spices. Our favourite combination is cardamom, black garlic, coriander and sea salt.

When preparing vegetables, if you're using organic vegetables such as carrots or parsnips you only need to rub the skin to get them clean; that way you keep much of the nutrition, which is in the skin. For non-organic vegetables, it's best to peel them.

Sourcing sustainable fish isn't always easy because it depends on how the fish is farmed or caught. You can ask your local fishmonger or supermarket about their own sustainability policy. The supplier we use has a 'sustainability and provenance' section for every fish or shellfish they sell on their website. The Marine Conservation Society is also an invaluable resource (www.fishonline.org).

For more information about ingredients, turn to the extra features throughout the book on sourcing meat (page 196), unusual ingredients (page 61), herbs and edible flowers (page 71), spices (page 82), grains (page 28) and seasonal ingredients (page 54).

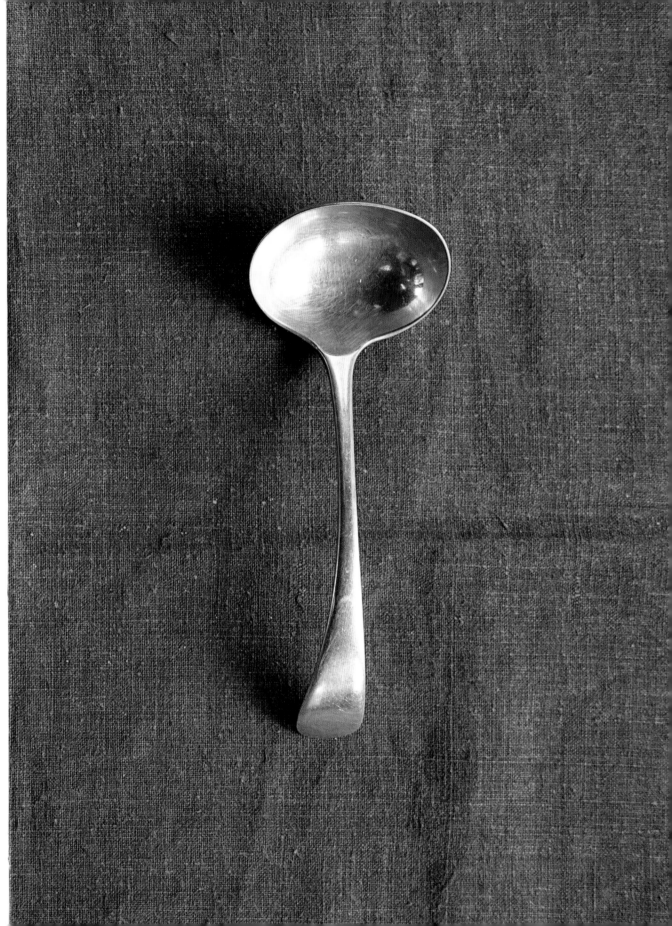

BEEF STOCK

MAKES 1 LITRE

1kg veal marrow bones
500g calves' feet
500g chicken wings
1 onion, quartered
1 leek, roughly chopped
1 celery stalk, roughly chopped
1 garlic clove

This is the essence of all kitchens. If you continue to reduce it on a low heat you will end up with the most wonderfully silky liquid that can be enjoyed on its own or with a little quinoa.

Preheat the oven to 210°C/fan 190°C/410°F/gas mark 7. Place the bones in a roasting tray and roast for 2–3 hours, until they are well coloured. Put the bones in a large pot with the calves' feet and chicken wings and cover with about 2 litres water.

Add the onion, leek, celery and garlic, bring to the boil and gently simmer on a very low heat for up to 8 hours. Strain the stock through a sieve lined with muslin and store in an airtight container in the refrigerator for up to a week (or freeze).

PRAWN STOCK

MAKES 1 LITRE

1kg raw prawn heads and shells
aromatics of your choice, such
   as lime zest, sweet chilli
   sauce, lemongrass, kaffir lime
   leaves or galangal
flaky sea salt

Don't be squeamish about using prawns heads for this stock as they hold most of the flavour.

Cover the prawn heads and your chosen aromatics with about 1.2 litres water, bring to the boil and reduce the heat to a simmer. Cook gently for 45 minutes, then strain. Taste to check the seasoning and store in the refrigerator for 2 days (or freeze). It makes a lovely base for prawn or shellfish soups.

SEAWEED & MUSHROOM STOCK

MAKES 1 LITRE

1 strip kombu seaweed
a handful of dried shiitake
   mushrooms
a small piece of fresh root
   ginger

This dashi-like stock makes a fantastic base for fish or noodle-based soups, and is so healthy.

Bring 1 litre water to the boil in a large pan, then allow it to cool. Once cool, add the kombu and leave it to soak for 10 minutes. Bring the liquid to a lively simmer, then reduce heat to a low simmer. Remove the kombu and add the dried shiitake mushrooms and fresh ginger, then continue to simmer gently for 30 minutes. Remove the ginger and discard it.

You can use the mushrooms for a stir-fry or keep them for a soup. This stock is best used on the same day, but it keeps for 2 days in an airtight container in the refrigerator (or you can freeze it).

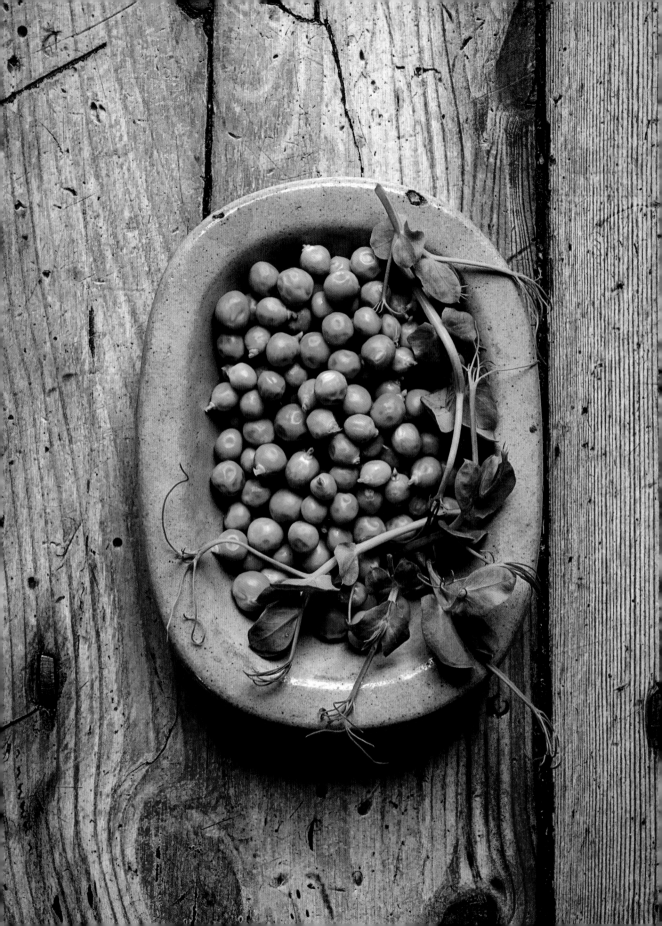

QUICK FIXES

The beauty of soup is that you can make it out of pretty much any ingredient you fancy

It's easy to convince ourselves that we don't have time to cook. By the time we get home from a long day, all we often want to do is flop on the sofa. These quick-fix recipes are the answer, as they're short on time but rich in flavour. In the time it takes to cook some noodles, you can raid your storecupboard or freezer and have a bowl of fresh and vibrant flavours on the table. That's why our cupboards are full of different varieties of rice, noodles (we especially love all the wheat-free varieties now available), lentils, pulses and grains. With a carton of passata and an onion you can turn a few humble chickpeas into a spicy Chana Masala, or make your life wholesome with some

farro (pearled spelt) and a bag of spinach to make Greens and Grains.

But don't stop with our ideas. The beauty of soup is that you can make it out of pretty much any ingredient you happen to fancy, along with your stock. And remember that things go a long way with soup, so if you only have a couple of rashers of bacon, you can chop them up and add them to a spicy dal, and some leftover chicken will look far more generous in a pot of broth, rice and vegetables than it will sitting lonely on a plate. The by-product of actually spending 10 minutes in the kitchen is that it does work as a form of relaxation or winding down. Everyone loves a quick fix.

CALDO VERDE

SERVES 2

½ tbsp unsalted butter
½ onion, finely chopped
1 garlic clove, crushed
½ tbsp olive oil
1 leek, halved lengthways, thinly sliced
1 potato, cut into 1cm cubes
½ tsp paprika
600ml hot vegetable or chicken stock (pages 14–15)
½ tbsp tomato purée
50g cooking chorizo, cut into 1cm cubes
50g kale, hard stems removed, leaves shredded
extra-virgin olive oil, to serve
flaky sea salt

Kate discovered this soup when she was looking up what to make with the food that was left over in the fridge: a couple of potatoes, some kale, a leek and some chorizo sausage. It turns out that's just what you need to make a quick-fix *caldo verde* ('green broth' in Portuguese).

Melt the butter in a heavy-based pan, add the onion and cook gently for a few minutes before adding the garlic. Add the olive oil and then the leek, and continue to cook for about 5 minutes, or until soft. Add the potato, season with salt, add the paprika and cook, stirring well, for a couple of minutes.

Add the hot stock and tomato purée, bring to the boil, reduce the heat to a simmer and cook gently until the potatoes are almost tender, around 5–15 minutes, depending on the type of potato.

Heat a small frying pan and add the chorizo; it has enough of its own fat so you don't need to add any more to the pan. Fry it until slightly crispy, then set aside.

Add the shredded kale to the stock and vegetables and cook for about 5 minutes, until just tender. Season with salt to taste. Ladle into bowls and top with the chorizo and a drizzle of extra-virgin olive oil.

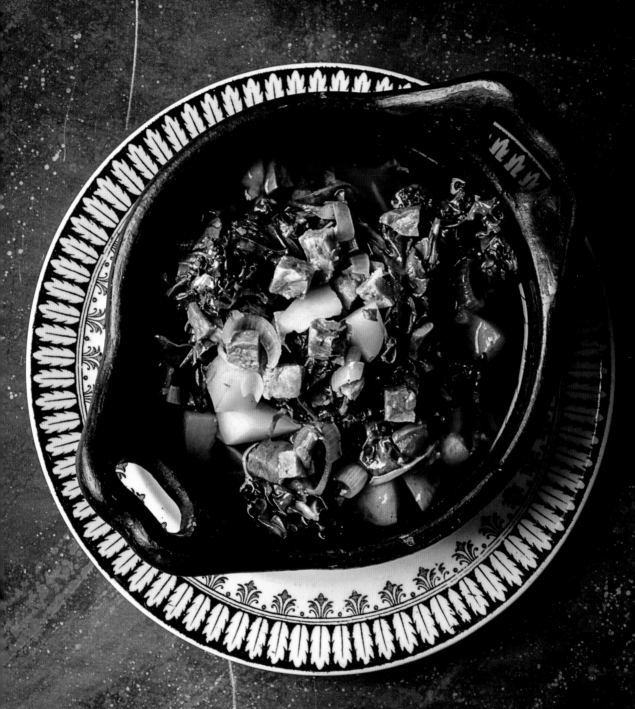

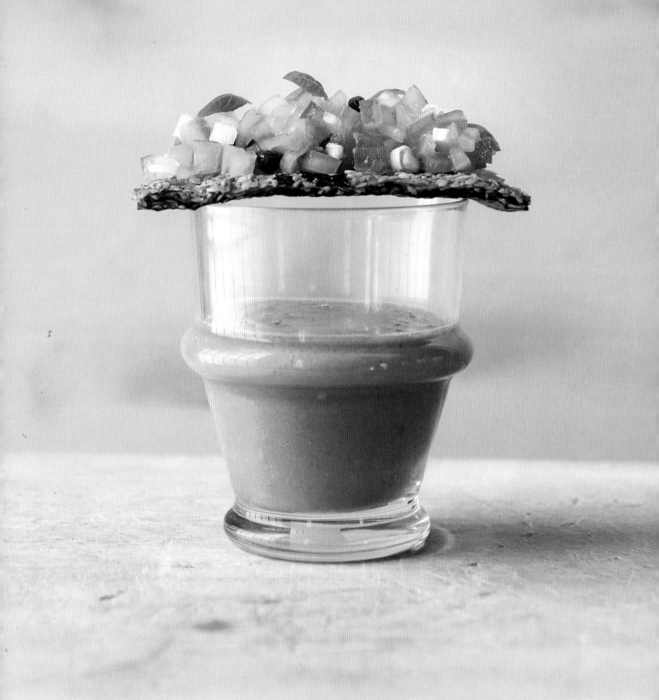

ROASTED CHERRY TOMATO SOUP WITH SALSA & FLATBREADS

SERVES 2

500g mixed heritage or cherry
    tomatoes, on the vine
1 tbsp olive oil
1 tbsp balsamic vinegar
1 tsp grated unwaxed lemon zest
1/2 tbsp capers, rinsed, drained
    and chopped
1 spring onion, thinly sliced
200ml hot vegetable stock
    (page 15)
1 tbsp tomato purée
flaky sea salt
seeded flatbreads, to serve

Tomatoes were rather boring in the UK for many years. They all looked the same, and as a result tasted of very little. Things are greatly improving, thanks to farmers' markets, farm shops and people growing their own. This tomato soup is very summery and aromatic; tomatoes on the vine have a distinctive smell that goes so well with the lemon zest and capers.

Preheat the oven to 230°C/fan 210°C/450°F/gas mark 8. Arrange 400g of the tomatoes in a single layer on a baking sheet. Drizzle with the olive oil and balsamic vinegar, sprinkle with the lemon zest and season with salt. Roast for about 10 minutes, until the tomatoes are bursting and soft. Now switch off the oven and allow the tomatoes to soften in the residual heat.

Meanwhile, to make the salsa, chop the remaining cherry tomatoes and mix them with the capers and spring onion.

Remove the roasted cherry tomatoes from the vines and put them in a blender with the hot stock and tomato purée. Blend until smooth. Serve with the salsa and seeded flatbreads.

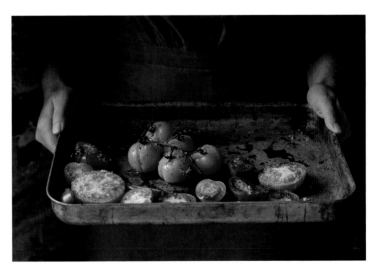

WATERCRESS SOUP WITH CRAB TOASTS

SERVES 4

1 tbsp unsalted butter
1 onion, chopped
1 medium potato, diced
850ml chicken stock (page 14)
400g watercress, rinsed
a little unsweetened almond
    milk or water, if needed
flaky sea salt and freshly
    ground black pepper
ready-made fresh crab pâté
    and pumpkin seed crackers
    (we like Dr Karg's), to serve

Our friend, medicine woman, Emma Cannon tells us that according to traditional Chinese medicine, watercress is excellent for the liver, which makes this a de-stressing, detoxing soup. Our top tip is to separate the watercress leaves from the stalks, so you can lightly cook the stalks and then add the leaves raw, just before blending. It's definitely worth it for the intense watercress flavour and incredibly rich green colour.

Melt the butter in a large saucepan, add the onion and cook gently for a few minutes, stirring, until soft. Add the potato and cook for a few minutes more, then add the stock. Bring to the boil and reduce the heat to a simmer and cook for around 15 minutes, or until the potato is cooked.

Meanwhile, pick the watercress leaves from the stalks and set aside. Add the stalks to the pan 5 minutes before the potatoes have finished cooking, so that they just wilt.

Take the soup off the heat and add the watercress leaves, then process to a smooth consistency in a blender. Season with salt and pepper to taste. Add a little almond milk or water, if needed, to loosen it to your desired consistency. Serve with fresh crab pâté on pumpkin seed crackers.

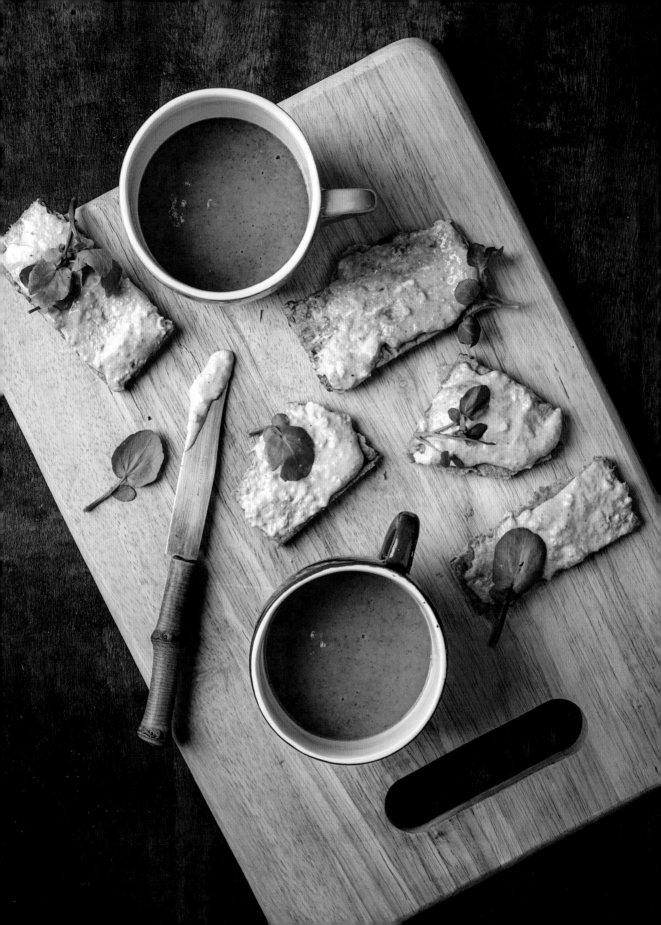

GREENS & GRAINS

SERVES 2

1 tsp olive oil

2 tbsp quinoa

400ml hot vegetable or
   chicken stock (pages 14–15)

100g farro (or other grain, such
   as pearl barley or freekeh)

2 large handfuls of kale (or
   other leafy greens, such
   as cavolo nero, spinach or
   rainbow chard), hard stems
   removed, leaves shredded

2 tbsp tahini

lemon juice, to taste

2 tbsp toasted flaked almonds

2 tbsp pomegranate seeds

red amaranth or purple shiso
   (optional)

This soup looks a picture, but it's very quick and easy to prepare. We love how tahini becomes creamy and light just by whisking in a little water and lemon juice. If you don't have pomegranate seeds to hand, this is the type of recipe you can easily adapt by adding seeds, toasted pine nuts or hazelnuts, a few sultanas or dried blueberries or cranberries.

Heat the oil in a large pan, add the quinoa and toast it for a minute or so until golden, shaking the pan frequently. Add the hot stock and farro, bring to the boil and simmer until tender (about 10 minutes if semi-pearled; check the packet instructions, as cooking times vary).

Turn off the heat, add the kale and leave it to sit until wilted. Mix the tahini with a little water and a squeeze of lemon juice until it becomes hummus-like in consistency. Ladle the soup into bowls and top with the kale and tahini sauce, then sprinkle with a scattering of toasted almonds, pomegranate seeds and, if using, red amaranth or purple shiso.

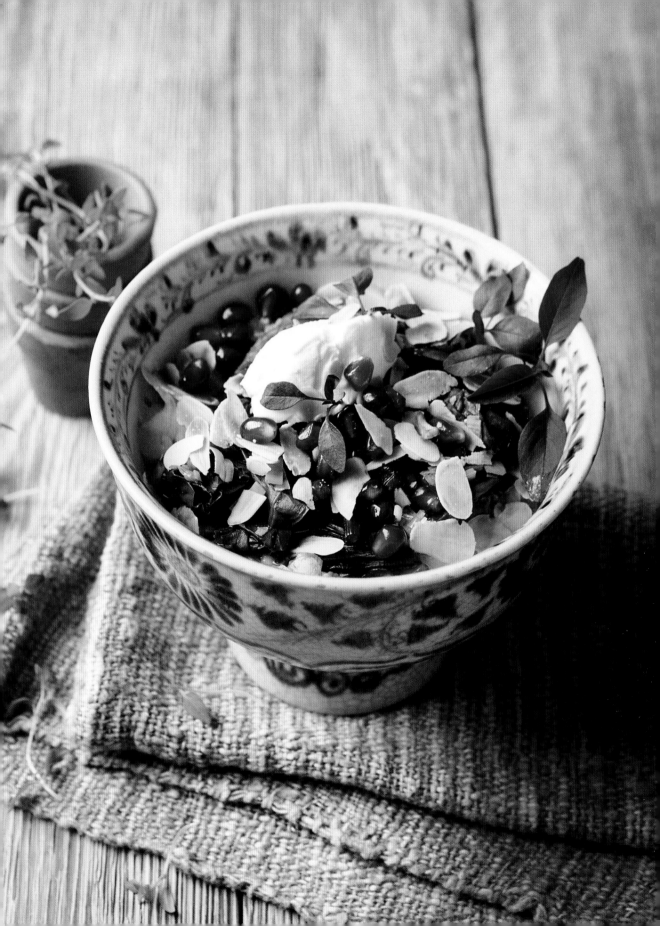

GREAT GRAINS
& SUPER SEEDS

We aim for most of our soups to be the main event of a meal, so we often use grains and seeds and have discovered some very interesting and delicious varieties. They are becoming increasingly available to buy, too; we thought freekeh was something you could only find in specialist shops until we spotted it in a local supermarket. Here are some of our favourites.

Amaranth: You'll probably have to search for amaranth, which is technically a seed, in your local health-food shop rather than in the supermarket. It's gluten free and high in protein and calcium. It was grown by the Aztecs in South America and is still a native crop of Peru, while in Asia it is often the leaves that are used in cooking. (See Ancient Amaranth, page 115.)

Buckwheat: Like amaranth, buckwheat is also a seed, despite its name, which makes it a great grain alternative if you follow a gluten-free diet. It's also a good source of fibre and contains some protein. It's slightly nutty in flavour and hearty in soups, and therefore perfect for autumn and winter. Even its flowers are loved by honey bees, so it's all good! (See Carrot and Roasted Buckwheat, page 105.)

Farro (or Emmer): Farro is an ancient wheat, so although it does contain gluten, it is less mass-produced than some wheat varieties. We are not sensitive to gluten but we do like to include a variety of grains to benefit our general digestive health. For a quick soup, pearled farro only takes 10–20 minutes to cook, while whole farro can take up to an hour. (See Greens and Grains, page 26, and Hot Cucumber, page 72.)

Freekeh: This grain is traditionally grown in the Middle East, and is made from wheat that is harvested early, hence its slightly green colour. The husk is removed by roasting the grain, and the result is quite a large grain that maintains its bite and goes particularly well with big flavours, like those from the Middle East such as cumin, coriander and sumac or pomegranate seeds. It's packed with B vitamins, which help us turn carbohydrates into energy, heading off afternoon slumps at the pass. (See Carrot, Cumin and Miso with Freekeh, page 51.)

Polenta: Made from corn, polenta is another gluten-free food that is very quick and convenient to make. Kate was a bit wary of making polenta, thinking it must be complicated to get that lovely, smooth consistency, but it's really very simple. You might assume that it needs lots of Parmesan cheese to taste good, but it actually has a sweet, savoury flavour of its own, so often all it needs is a little milk, water and sea salt. We've used it in our Mussels and Polenta recipe (page 184), and it's also delicious with balsamic mushrooms, or with steak or a stew, plus you can use it to make delicious gluten-free cakes.

Quinoa (pronounced 'keen-wah'): Like amaranth, quinoa is a seed traditionally grown in South America. You can now find black quinoa and red quinoa, which, like darker rice varieties, seem a bit more rugged but are equally delicious. Both amaranth and quinoa benefit from a quick chef's tip, which is to toast them for a minute in a dry pan before adding water, so that they keep a little bite. When the quinoa is cooked, drain any excess liquid, then cover it with a cloth to help the grains puff up and separate. Quinoa contains no gluten, so it's a good alternative to couscous and bulgur wheat. However, it's thought that those with coeliac disease may be sensitive to some of its proteins in a similar way to gluten. (See Marrow Soup with Courgette Flowers and Pesto Quinoa, page 176.)

Rice: White rice gets a bit of bad press for being a 'refined' food, and it's true that many of the nutrients are stripped in the polishing process that makes it white. However, when you're feeling under the weather or very stressed, your body will thank you for cooking up a batch of Congee (see page 109), which is so easy on the digestion and builds your appetite as you eat. We love the many varieties of rice you can now find, from brown to red, wild or black rice. These less processed varieties contain more fibre and break down into energy more gradually. (See also Cima di Rapa, page 62 and Green Tea, Brown Rice, page 76.)

Pumpkin seeds: These often add the perfect element of crunch to a soup (see Winter Miso, page 80 and Courgette and Za'atar, page 31). They contain a lot of nutrients and antioxidants, plus good fats, which is why they are a healthy snack to have around.

Sesame seeds: We love to sprinkle white or black sesame seeds on soups, especially any Asian recipes. Furikake is a brilliant Asian seasoning made with both types of sesame seed and seaweed flakes (see Resources, page 231). They're only small, but sesame seeds are packed with minerals and are always worth having in the cupboard.

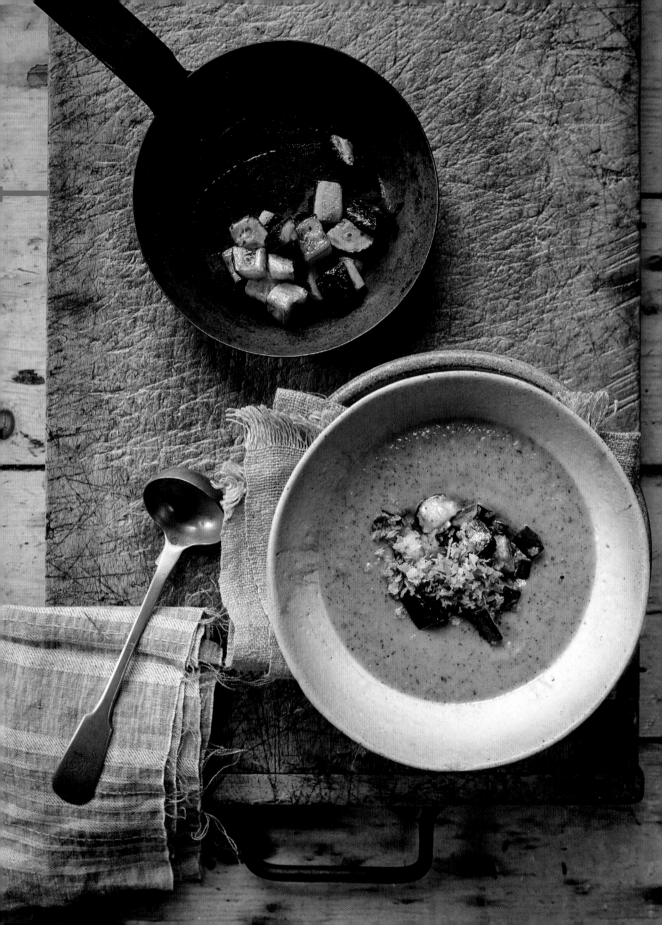

COURGETTE & ZA'ATAR

SERVES 4

4 tbsp light olive oil
600g courgettes (about 6),
    cut into cubes
3 tsp za'atar (page 82)
600ml hot chicken or
    vegetable stock (pages 14–15)
4 tbsp panko or dried
    breadcrumbs
1 tbsp fresh lemon thyme,
    leaves picked and chopped
1 tsp flaky sea salt

The idea for this soup came from roasting vegetables in the spice mix za'atar, a blend of wild thyme, sesame seeds, olive oil and sumac. In summer, courgettes grow like mad, and this is a quick way of putting a bag of them to delicious use. Panko breadcrumbs are becoming increasingly available in supermarkets as well as Asian stores. We love them because they are so light and fluffy.

Heat half the oil in a heavy-based pan and cook the courgettes gently for about 3 minutes. Stir in the za'atar.

Add the hot stock, bring to the boil, then reduce the heat to a simmer and cook gently until the courgettes are cooked but not too soft. Taste to check they're the consistency you like.

In the meantime, heat the remaining oil in a shallow pan and gently fry the panko crumbs, lemon thyme and salt, stirring frequently, until the breadcrumbs are golden and crisp.

Remove the courgettes from the heat and allow to cool slightly before processing half of them in a blender, using as much stock from the pan as you need to reach the desired consistency. Divide the remaining courgettes among 4 bowls in a pyramid shape, then gently ladle in the blended soup around the courgettes. Add a generous sprinkle of fried breadcrumbs to each bowl, then serve.

CAULIFLOWER SOUP
WITH DUKKAH

SERVES 4

1 cauliflower
1 tbsp unsalted butter
1 heaped tsp dukkah (page 82),
    plus extra to serve
600–750ml unsweetened
    almond milk
flaky sea salt and freshly
    ground black pepper
sesame oil, to serve (optional)
1 lemon, for squeezing
    (optional)
winter savoury herb, to garnish
    (optional)

Cauliflower and the spice blend dukkah (page 82) are a perfect match. Try experimenting with different kinds of dukkah: you can buy dukkah with 80 per cent hazelnut or a spicy version. Dukkah is one of our favourite toppings, we like to add it to scrambled eggs or dip fruit into it. If you've ever thought cauliflower is bland or boring, make this soup. We have never been disappointed.

Cut the cauliflower into small pieces, reserving a few thinly sliced florets for the garnish. Heat the butter in a wok or deep-sided frying pan, add the cauliflower and cook, stirring constantly, for a few minutes. This helps to release the flavour.

Add the dukkah and continue to cook for 2 more minutes before adding enough almond milk to cover the cauliflower. Bring to the boil and simmer for about 10 minutes, or until the cauliflower is cooked. Process in a blender and serve with a drizzle of sesame oil, a squeeze of lemon juice, the reserved cauliflower slices, some winter savoury, if using, and a little more dukkah sprinkled on top.

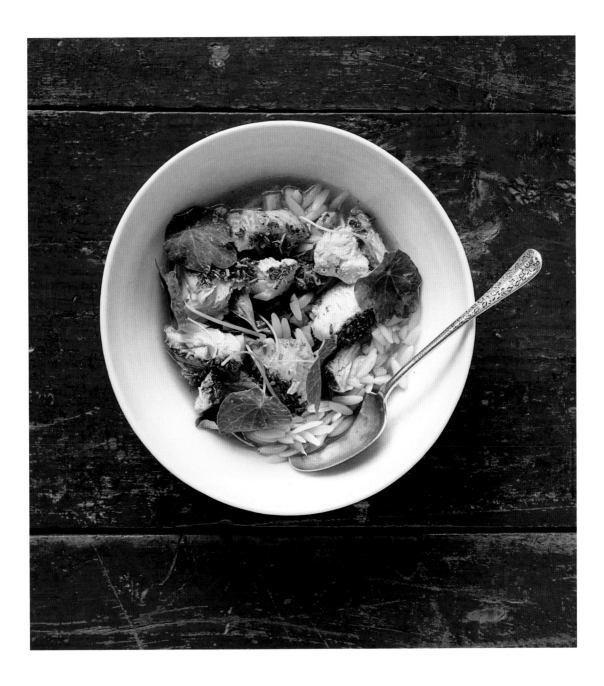

SALMON & ORZO

SERVES 2

1 tsp fennel seeds

zest of 1 unwaxed lemon, in strips

1 tsp sumac

2 salmon fillets, about 150g each

1 tsp wholegrain mustard

100g orzo pasta

400ml chicken stock (page 14)

1 baby gem lettuce, shredded

20g fresh dill, finely chopped

extra-virgin olive oil, to dress
  the leaves

flaky sea salt

a handful of nasturtium leaves
  or pea shoots, to serve
  (optional)

We treat fish in the same way as meat, now that we've learned a little more about where it comes from and how sustainable it is. We're eating less of it, but buying it from good sources. The combination of salmon with orzo pasta, peas and baby gem lettuce in this soup are very pleasing for a mid-week treat.

Preheat the oven to 140°C/fan 120°C/275°F/gas mark 1.

Spread out the fennel seeds and lemon zest on an oven tray and dry-roast in the oven for 10–15 minutes. Tip into a pestle and mortar and grind to a powder, stirring in the sumac.

Increase the oven temperature to 230°C/fan 210°C/450°F/gas mark 8. Brush the salmon fillets with mustard, then evenly scatter over the fennel, zest and sumac mixture. Bake for about 8 minutes, until the flesh can be flaked, but is still soft and dark pink in the middle. Set aside and let rest.

Meanwhile, cook the orzo pasta in boiling water until al dente (check the packet instructions for the timing), then drain. Heat the chicken stock and tip the orzo into the stock. Toss the baby gem lettuce and dill in a little extra-virgin olive oil and sea salt. Ladle the orzo broth into bowls and top with the salmon, baby gem, dill, salmon and a few nasturtium leaves or pea shoots to serve.

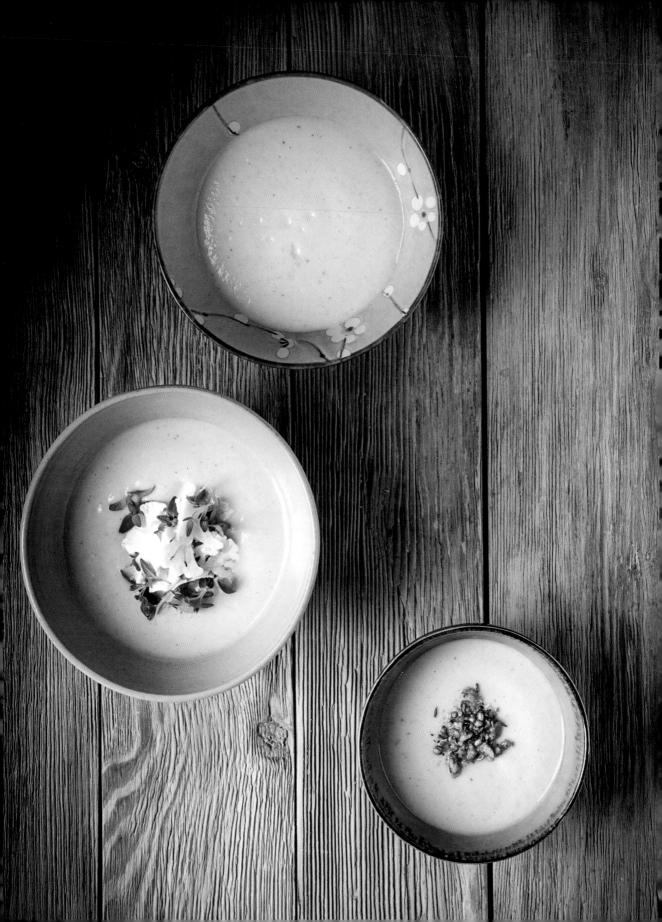

DROP AN EGG

SERVES 2

80g fresh shiitake mushrooms
1 tbsp olive oil
400ml hot chicken or
   vegetable stock (pages 14–15)
1 tsp cornflour
½ tsp grated fresh root ginger
1 tbsp tamari (soy) sauce
2 eggs
2 spring onions, thinly sliced

We believe the world would be a duller place without eggs. They provide excellent protein that will keep you fuller for longer, while shiitake mushrooms, spring onions and fresh ginger are all super-healthy too. This is such a simple but satisfying soup.

Preheat the oven to 230°C/fan 210°C/450°F/gas mark 8. Remove the tough stalks from the mushrooms, finely slice them, then mix them with the olive oil in a large bowl. Place in a baking dish and roast for about 10 minutes, until soft.

Combine 50ml of the hot stock with the cornflour to make a smooth paste. Put the remaining stock in a saucepan with the ginger, tamari and roasted shiitake and bring to the boil. Add the stock-cornflour mixture and reduce the heat to a simmer, stirring.

Beat the eggs in a small bowl, then slowly pour them into the soup, so that it turns into threads on impact as it cooks. Scatter over the spring onions before serving. We like to eat Vegemite, mascarpone and cucumber sandwiches with this soup.

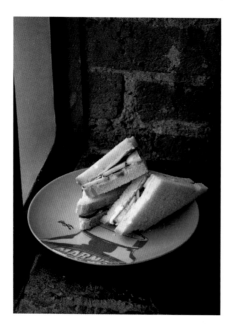

CHANA MASALA

SERVES 2

1 tbsp olive oil
1 onion, finely chopped
½ tsp garam masala
½ tsp ground turmeric
½ tsp ground ginger
¼ tsp chilli flakes
300g tomato passata
1 x 400g tin chickpeas, rinsed
    and drained
200ml tinned coconut milk
flaky sea salt
Greek yoghurt, to serve

This is a quick and easy spicy soup supper, perfect for a Meatless Monday (a campaign that began in the US, designed to encourage and inspire people to eat less meat for the good of the planet). We're both meat lovers, and are unlikely to go vegetarian or vegan very soon, but we do love the concept of Meatless Mondays. We're always looking for delicious vegetarian dishes, and spices can really bring simple ingredients to life.

Heat the oil in a heavy-based pan, add the onion and cook gently for about 10 minutes or until soft and translucent. Add the spices and cook, stirring, until the aromas are released. After a couple of minutes, add the tomato passata, chickpeas and coconut milk. Bring to just below boiling point and simmer gently for 30 minutes to help the flavours develop. Season with salt and serve with spoonfuls of Greek yoghurt.

ALL IN THE DETAIL

A great deal of a chef's work consists of quietly and calmly getting on with prep, in other words, chopping and preparing vegetables, aromatics and base ingredients for hours at a time. We don't see this side of the kitchen on reality television shows, where everything is focused on the performance and drama of the last moments of a dish. From Nicole, Kate learned the importance of chopping vegetables finely to make a *mirepoix*: in other words, the chopped onion, celery and carrot that so often forms the base of soups. She then discovered that in Italy this is called the *soffritto*, and that in almost every cuisine there are two or three ingredients that provide the underlying foundation for the main flavours to build upon. Soups often need a simpler but more detailed approach than most grilled or roasted dishes; they don't clamour for our attention, but do give a great deal of satisfaction.

Watch a chef in the kitchen and you will often see a person in complete flow. Kate always thinks they work so much harder than others in many professions but she also envies their ability to be present in the moment, to be gently and expertly focused on what they are doing rather than constantly looking around for the next distraction. Chefs teach us to celebrate the importance of the details, such as letting your meat rest and relax; chopping finely, which means *really* finely; tasting everything before you season; choosing your bowls with care; and keeping your knives sharp.

We have also learned that garnishes matter, because these add that bit of crunch, creaminess or flavour that brings a dish together. It's worth scattering over a few bright, fresh herbs, or drizzling over a little good extra-virgin olive oil, a handful of toasted seeds and nuts, some crumbled feta marinated in mustard and caraway seeds that were quickly fried in olive oil until they popped, or a dollop of Greek yoghurt or crème fraîche mixed with grated lime zest. Show your soups some love and attention with these small details and they will repay you for it.

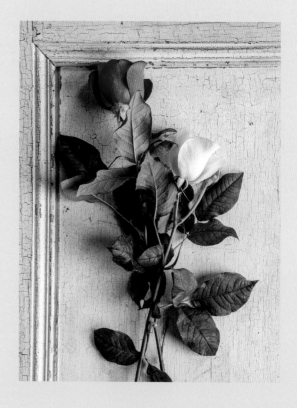

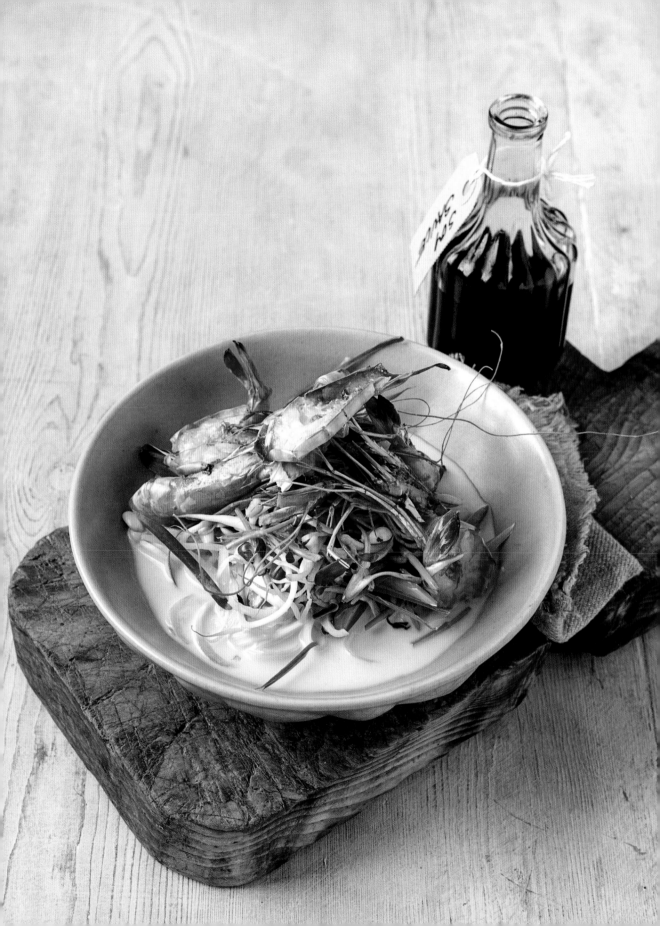

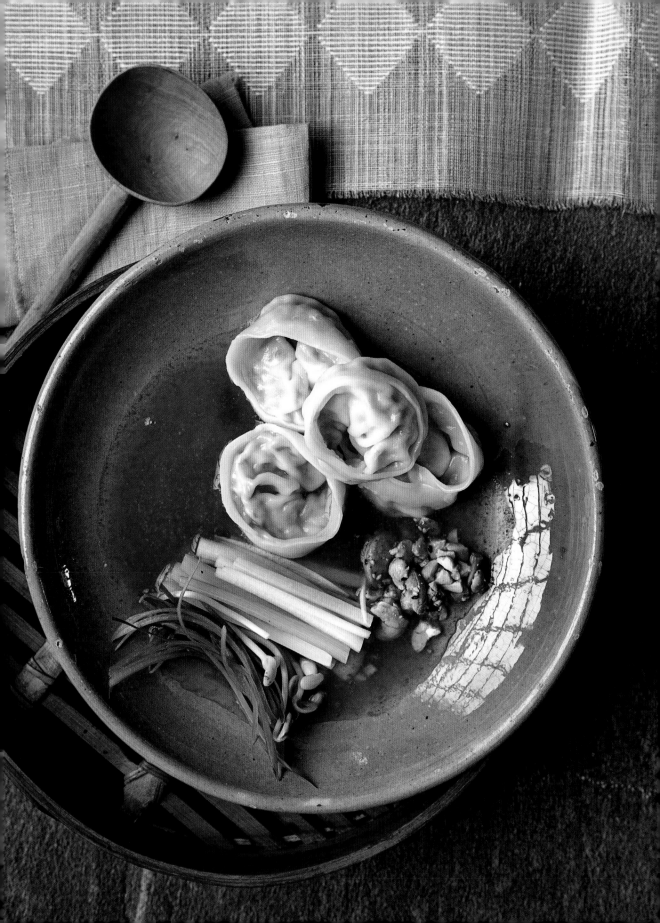

SOHO DUMPLINGS

SERVES 2

8–10 (about 200g) ready-made
    gyoza
400ml chicken, vegetable or
    seaweed and mushroom
    stock (pages 14, 15 and 17)
1 tbsp Thai chilli paste
1 celery stalk, thinly sliced
    lengthways
few handfuls beansprouts
2 spring onions, thinly sliced
    lengthways
2 tbsp cashew nuts, toasted
    and crushed
flaky sea salt

This is inspired by our favourite Chinese dumpling café in Soho, London, where the dumplings are made fresh in the window. A friend of ours makes her own gyoza, which makes for very impressive dinner parties. For this quick fix, though, you can buy them ready-made from most supermarkets or Asian stores.

Cook the gyoza according to the instructions on the packet.

To make the soup, heat the stock in a saucepan. Loosen the Thai chilli paste with a little stock before adding it to the pan along with the celery. Bring to the boil, then reduce the heat to a simmer and cook for 3–4 minutes. Season to taste with sea salt. Divide the gyoza among the bowls. Ladle over the hot broth and add a handful of beansprouts to each bowl, followed by the spring onions and cashew nuts. Serve immediately.

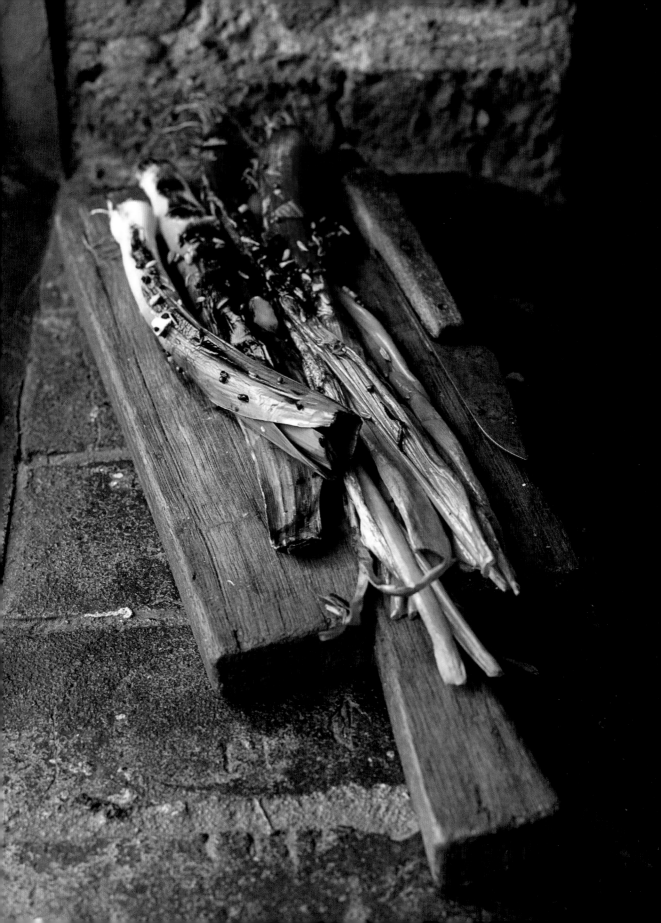

ROOTS & TUBERS

Just when we thought we had our five-a-day sorted,
we discover that we're supposed to try and eat nine
portions of fruit and veg every day!

Most of us are looking for easy and delicious ways to get more vegetables into our diet. Just when we thought we had our five-a-day sorted, we discover that we're supposed to try and eat nine portions of fruit and veg every day! There's only so much green juice we can take, so vegetable soups are the way to go.

Roots and tubers are some of the most versatile vegetables around when it comes to creating satisfying, tasty soups. Carrots will happily meld with ginger, orange, coriander, cumin or miso (try our Carrot, Cumin and Miso Soup with Freekeh) and squash likes all of these flavours, as well as chilli, cinnamon and coconut (as shown in Butternut Squash and Caramelised Pear). A good beetroot soup, like Beetroot and Burrata, tastes as though it will nourish you for a week. When you gently simmer or roast root vegetables, they become wonderfully easy to digest, making their range of nutrients easier for our bodies to absorb. Perhaps that's why they're so satisfying.

CELERIAC MIMOSA

SERVES 4

1 tbsp unsalted butter
1 celeriac, peeled and roughly
    diced
750ml hot chicken or vegetable
    stock (pages 14–15)
250ml unsweetened rice or
    almond milk
2 eggs
1/2 stick celery, finely chopped
flaky sea salt

If you go by looks alone you might never pick up a celeriac. A humble vegetable with a glorious taste, it has a good depth of flavour with all the pleasant taste of celery and gives a creamy texture.

Melt the butter in a large saucepan, add the celeriac and cook gently until it starts to soften. Add the stock and milk to cover and simmer gently for about 15 minutes, or until soft. Process the soup in a blender until smooth, then taste and season with salt.

Meanwhile, boil the eggs for 8 minutes, cool them under running water, then peel and chop them. Stir in the chopped celery, season with salt, and serve with the soup.

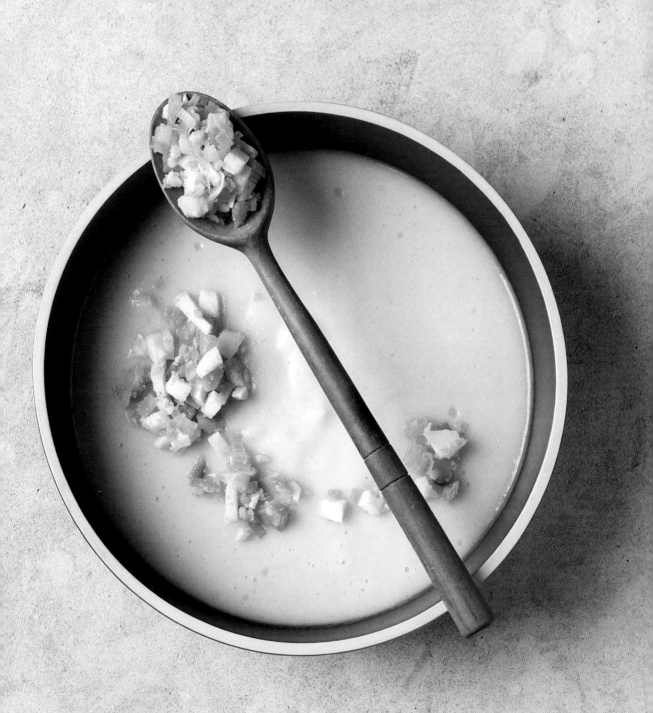

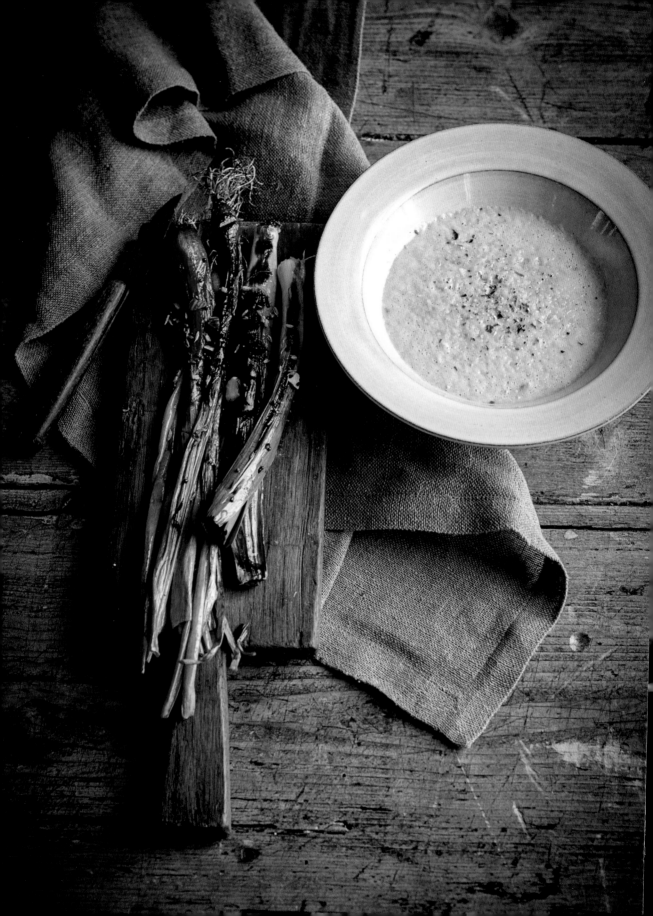

LEEK & NEW POTATO SOUP WITH CALÇOTS

SERVES 2

2 leeks

2 tsp unsalted butter

4 small new potatoes, quartered

300ml soya milk

1 tsp black onion seeds, plus
    extra to serve

zest of 1/2 unwaxed lemon,
    finely grated

4 calçot onions

olive oil, for the onions

flaky sea salt and freshly
    ground black pepper

Calçots are a type of long, sweet-tasting onion, grown in Spain where they are in season from late November to March, and at the *Gran Fiesta de la Calçotada* in Valls each January, thousands of people gather to talk and eat onions. It's great to explore different ingredients, and not be afraid of vegetables you haven't seen before. If you can't find calçots, baby leeks or red salad onions are good alternatives. You'll need a ridged grill pan to produce the best flavour from the onions.

Cut the leeks in half lengthways and slice the pale green parts, discarding the tough outer dark-green leaves.

Melt half the butter in a saucepan, add the leeks and cook for a few minutes until they soften, then add the potatoes. Mix the soya milk, black onion seeds and lemon zest together and add to the vegetables. Bring to the boil, then reduce the heat to a simmer and cook for about 15 minutes, or until you can pierce the potatoes easily with a sharp knife. Process the soup in a blender until smooth, season with salt and pepper before returning it to the pan while you prepare the calçots.

To cook the calçots, heat a ridged grill pan. Wash them, brush them with olive oil and cook over a medium heat for 4–5 minutes until soft and slightly caramelised. Once they have cooled a little, pull back the outer layers to reveal the sweet centre. Divide the soup between 2 bowls and serve with the calçots on the side.

JERUSALEM ARTICHOKE

SERVES 4

800g Jerusalem artichokes
a little lemon juice
1 tbsp unsalted butter
750ml hot vegetable stock
    (page 15)
250ml whole milk
flaky sea salt

Nicole used to run a family restaurant in Malta, where she would cook food for the local orphanage. The orphanages were all run by nuns, and one day the nuns came to the restaurant to ask very nicely that she never make 'that artichoke soup' for them again. Nicole felt terrible, but couldn't help seeing the funny side. After all, however delicious artichoke soup is, it does tend to have an rather unfortunate consequence.

Scrub the artichokes and soak them for a couple of hours in cold water with a little lemon juice (this is thought to reduce that embarrassing side-effect of eating Jerusalem artichokes – fingers crossed!). Chop them roughly. Melt the butter in a pan, add the artichokes, season with salt, and cook gently for a few minutes. Add the hot stock and milk to cover. Bring to a simmer and cook for 10–15 minutes, or until the artichokes are soft. Process in a blender until smooth, then taste to check the seasoning. This soup is lovely with an oatcake, some ricotta and a few roasted hazelnuts.

YAM & COCONUT

SERVES 4

600g yams or sweet potatoes,
    peeled and cut into 2cm
    cubes
400ml tinned coconut milk
4 tbsp sweet chilli sauce
1 tbsp fish sauce (or soy sauce
    for a vegetarian alternative)
flaky sea salt

Purple or pale-fleshed yams are great for this soup, but they can be hard to find. Sweet potatoes work well, too. Yams always need to be peeled and cooked, as they can contain toxins.

Put the yams in a large saucepan with the coconut milk, bring almost to the boil, then reduce the heat to a simmer and cook for about 15 minutes, until tender. Remove from the pan and set aside.

Stir the sweet chilli sauce and fish sauce into the cooking liquid and season with salt, to taste. Process the cooked yams and cooking liquid in batches in a blender until smooth, then serve.

CARROT, CUMIN & MISO SOUP WITH FREEKEH

SERVES 4

For the soup
1 tbsp unsalted butter
1 onion, sliced
1 heaped tsp cumin seeds
1 kg carrots, roughly chopped
1 heaped tsp white miso paste

For the freekeh
100g freekeh, spelt or pearl
   barley
25g dried cranberries
¼ onion, finely chopped
½ celery stalk, finely chopped
½ carrot, finely chopped
flaky sea salt

In this recipe we've substituted miso for stock, since it combines well with the sweet carrots and spicy cumin. Freekeh is a type of wholegrain wheat (see page 28). It has a wonderful smoky aroma and flavour, and is slightly green in colour as it is harvested early. Like quinoa, it's rich in protein and makes this simple carrot soup into a hearty meal.

Melt the butter in a large pan, add the onion and cook for 10 minutes until soft. Push the onion to one side to create space in the pan and add the cumin seeds. When the seeds start to release their aroma, add the carrots and give everything a good stir. Add the miso paste and stir it through the vegetables, then add 750ml just-boiled water from the kettle. Bring to the boil, then simmer for 10 minutes, or until the carrots can be pierced with a sharp knife. Process the soup in a blender until smooth and season with salt.

To make the freekeh, put the grains in a pan, cover with water and bring to the boil. Simmer until the grains are cooked – about 45 minutes for freekeh, but check the instructions on the packet.

Meanwhile, soak the cranberries in warm water. When the freekeh is cooked, drain it and mix it with the drained cranberries and onion, celery and carrot in a large bowl. Season with a little salt.

Process the soup in a blender until smooth, then serve topped with the freekeh.

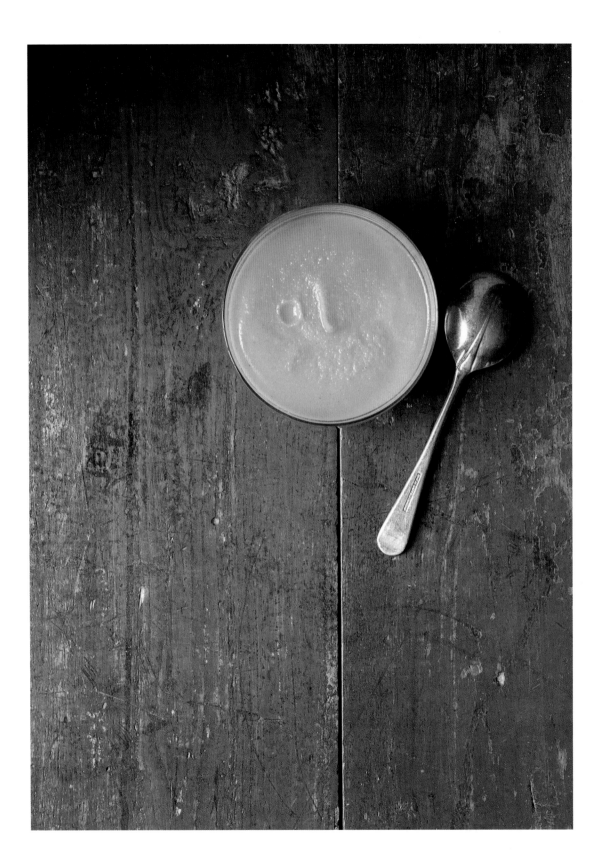

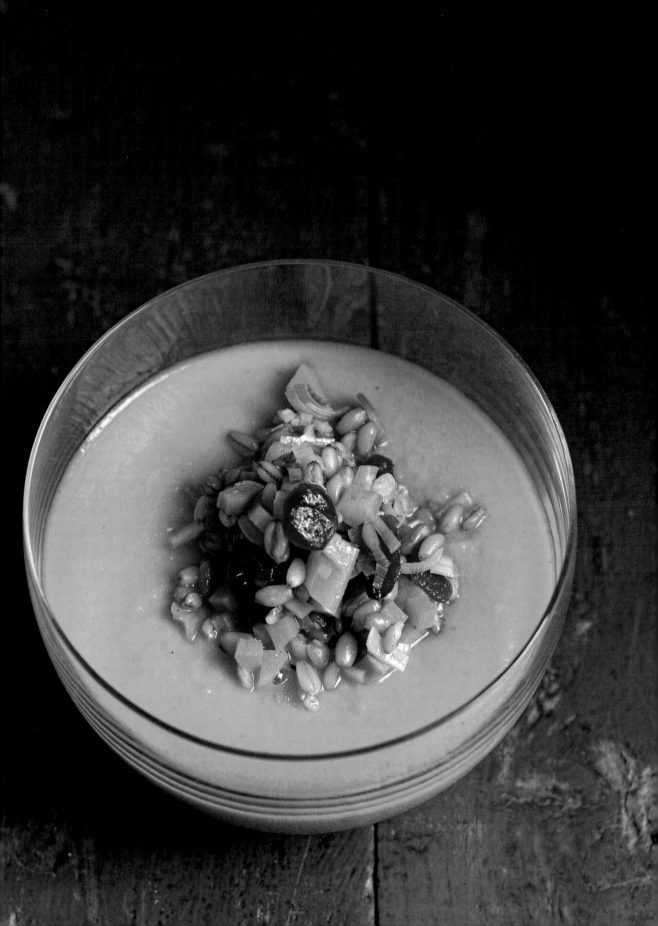

EAT WITH
THE SEASONS

Somehow, nature seems to provide the right foods at the right time. Just when our body needs warmth and comfort and we're happy to slow-cook a stew all Sunday long, root vegetables come into their own. When we feel the urge to eat lightly and cleanse our bodies, the leafy greens become bountiful and need only a little steaming. Eating seasonally goes hand in hand with eating a little more locally and discovering the vegetables, meat and fish that are available in our own region or country at particular times of the year. We search out the first English asparagus and Jersey Royal potatoes in spring, and we ask the fishmonger which fish came from our own shores and how fresh they are.

We're no experts, but we get to forage for the simple things in our gardens and down the lane; you can't miss the smell of wild garlic growing in the woods when you get near it, and when you snip your own nettle tops (leaving the rest for the caterpillars) to make soup (see page 69) or a simple fresh tea with the bright leaves, you know you're tasting spring. The colours of foods bring us the colours of the seasons: deep red tomatoes on a hot summer's day, earth-coloured mushrooms in autumn and winter; bright and fresh green leaves that burst through in the spring and deepen over the following months. When you eat with the seasons you eat with all your senses and feel at one with nature; this brings happiness.

Here is some of the seasonal produce to look out for and enjoy during the year. Any of these ingredients might span a couple of seasons; we're just giving a flavour of what is usually abundant at certain points during the cycle of the year.

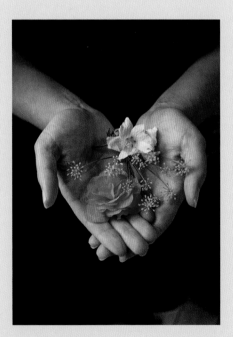

Winter warmth
beetroot
cauliflower
celeriac
chard
chicory
hazelnuts
horseradish
Jerusalem artichokes
kale
kohlrabi
leeks
parsnips
pomegranates
potatoes
swede
turnips
walnuts
wild mushrooms
winter cabbage

cod
mussels
scallop
salmon
venison

Spring cleanse
asparagus
broccoli
carrots
cauliflower
globe artichokes
Jersey Royals
kale
leeks
lettuce
nettles
radishes
rocket
spinach
spring cabbage
spring onions
sorrel
watercress
wild garlic

crab
prawns
sea trout
lamb

Summer joy
broad beans
carrots
courgettes
cucumber
edible flowers
fennel
French beans
globe artichokes
lettuce
new potatoes
peas
peppers
runner beans
sweetcorn
tomatoes

cod
crab
prawns
salmon
scallops

Autumn harvest
apples
aubergines
beetroot
carrots
courgettes
pears
pumpkin
squashes
wild mushrooms

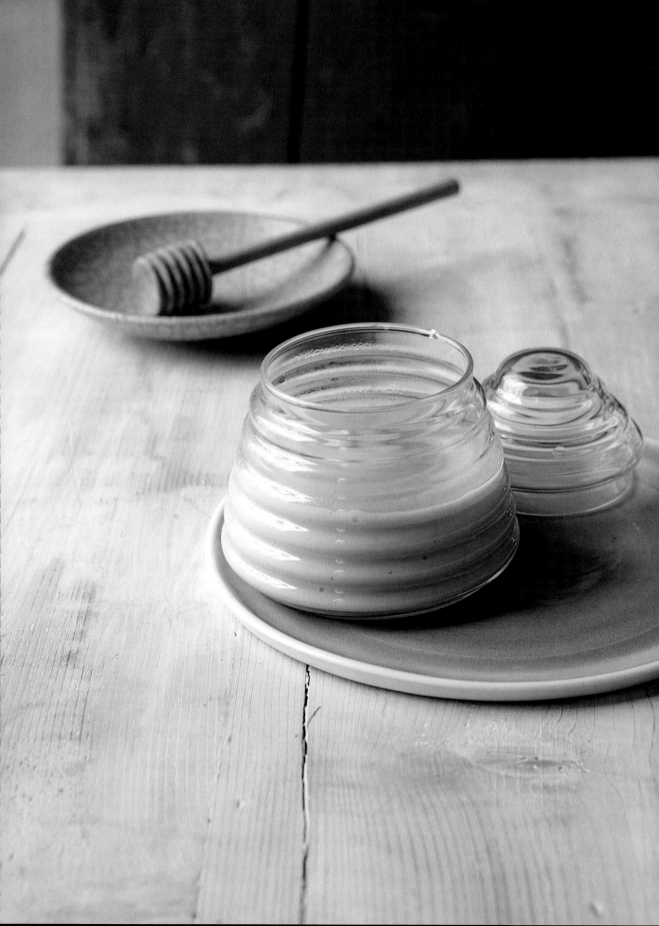

MANUKA HONEY PARSNIP

SERVES 4

1 tbsp unsalted butter
2 large parsnips, chopped
1 small swede, chopped
1 litre hot vegetable or chicken
    stock (pages 14–15)
3 tbsp manuka honey,
    or to taste
flaky sea salt and freshly
    ground black pepper

Root vegetables make a perfect soup for a winter's day. They take just minutes and we promise are so much better than shop bought; simple can be so good. We've used manuka honey for its extra goodness, but whichever honey you choose, go for raw honey when you can.

Melt the butter in a large pan, add the parsnips and swede and cook gently for a few minutes to release the flavour. Add the hot stock to cover. Bring to the boil, then reduce the heat to a simmer and cook for 15–20 minutes, until the vegetables are tender. Process the soup in a blender until smooth, season with salt and pepper and stir through the honey to taste.

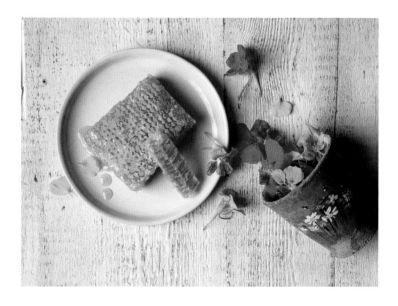

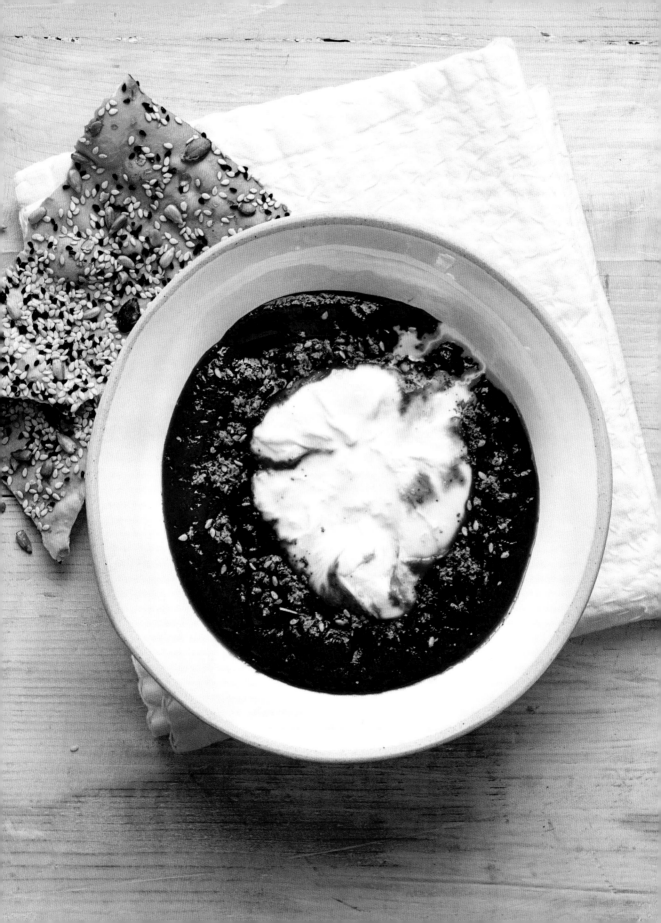

BEETROOT & BURRATA

SERVES 4

4 large beetroot, tops trimmed
   to about 2.5cm
1 tsp flaky sea salt
8 tbsp pomegranate vinegar
   (raspberry or balsamic
   vinegar will also work well)
1 tbsp fennel seeds
about 570ml whole milk
4 burrata or buffalo mozzarella
   cheeses, approximately
   125g each
flaky sea salt and freshly
   ground black pepper
seeded crackers, to serve

This soup is intense and quite wonderful. The pairing of beetroot with burrata, which is a type of creamy buffalo mozzarella, creates a perfect balance. It's a feast for all the senses, with the deep red contrasting against the white, and the aromas of sweet, vinegary beetroot roasting in your kitchen.

Preheat the oven to 190°C/fan 170°C/375°F/gas mark 5.

Place the beetroot in an ovenproof dish, sprinkle with salt and pour over the vinegar. Cover with foil and roast for about 1 1/2 hours, or until they can be easily pierced with a sharp knife. Remove and allow to cool. Turn the oven down to 140°C/fan 120°C/285°F/gas mark 1.

Sprinkle the fennel seeds on a baking tray and toast for about 10 minutes in the oven until aromatic.

If using organic beetroot, leave the skin on. If not, rub off the skin, preferably wearing kitchen gloves to avoid getting caught red-handed! Chop the beetroot roughly and process in a blender with enough milk to reach the desired consistency. Taste and season with salt and pepper if necessary.

Heat the soup gently in a pan, then serve in 4 bowls with a burrata for each person, a scattering of toasted fennel seeds and some seeded crackers.

SUMAC-ROASTED
SWEET POTATO

SERVES 4

800g sweet potatoes, roughly
    chopped (preferably white-
    fleshed, but orange is fine)
200g shallots, roughly chopped
4 tbsp olive oil
1 tbsp sumac, plus extra to serve
1 tsp flaky sea salt
1 litre vegetable or chicken
    stock (pages 14–15)
Greek yoghurt, to serve

Sumac is made from dried, blitzed sour berries. It is available in most supermarkets now, so we thought we'd celebrate with this simplest of soups. It has a smoky, almost citrusy aroma and a delicious, dark berry colour.

Preheat the oven to 200°C/180°C fan/400°F/gas mark 6.

In a large mixing bowl, thoroughly combine the sweet potatoes, shallots, olive oil, sumac and salt. Tip the vegetables into a large roasting tin (you might need two) and roast for about 15–20 minutes (for orange-fleshed sweet potatoes) or 30–45 minutes (for white-fleshed) until cooked. Halfway through cooking, give them a turn to prevent them from burning.

Allow to cool a little, then process in batches in a blender, adding some of the stock each time. Reheat the soup in a pan and serve with a spoonful of Greek yoghurt and a dusting of sumac.

FINDING THE UNUSUAL

You may find some unfamiliar ingredients within these pages, alongside the everyday ones. Like many chefs, Nicole seeks out new ingredients wherever she might be, whether it's discovering seaweed salt on the Isle of Skye or lily bulbs in Chinatown, just around the corner from work. She will spend hours wandering around the Japan Centre in London, but will also get lost in exploration in any supermarket, finding out which of the less commonplace ingredients are creating a significant enough trend to be embraced by the big brands.

Thanks to the growth of online food shops, every ingredient used in the recipes is at your fingertips, from kimchi kits to spices, unusual grains and edible flowers, and we have listed these in the Resources section (see page 231). Some of the ingredients are an occasional or seasonal treat for us – the nettles that grow in Kate's family's garden, for example, are fresh and bountiful for just a couple of months in spring – while other recently discovered ones have become storecupboard essentials, such as furikake (sesame seeds and seaweed), the perfect seasoning for almost any South Asian dish. We will happily sprinkle dukkah (a hazelnut spice blend) on eggs in the morning, roasted vegetables or grilled fish. Miso has become our third basic stock, alongside chicken and vegetable, and Nicole will reach for the quinoa as often as she'll think to use rice.

We hope the recipes provide inspiration to be on the look-out for interesting ingredients and soup ideas wherever you find yourself, whether you're discovering the local markets, eating the local dishes, or bringing the new tastes, sights and smells into your own kitchen.

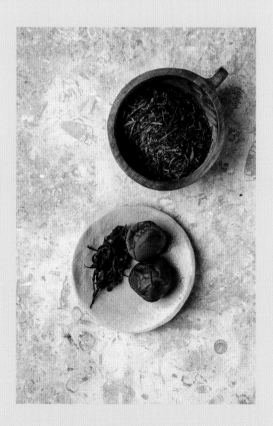

CIMA DI RAPA
WITH BLACK RICE AND OLIVES

SERVES 2

2 tbsp unsalted butter
1 onion, finely chopped
100g Thai black rice or wild
    rice, rinsed
600ml hot vegetable stock
    (page 15)
1 tsp wasabi paste
1 garlic clove, crushed
200g cima di rapa or broad
    bean tops, rinsed and
    shredded
flaky sea salt
seeded olive crackers, to serve

For the garnish
30g feta, crumbled
30g mixed olives, chopped
small handful turnip tops
3 tbsp extra-virgin olive oil,
    to serve

Cima di rapa is also less romantically known as turnip tops. We don't tend to use the tops of vegetables but this recipe makes great use of them. This soup is a fusion of Thai, Japanese and Mediterranean influences, yet everything works together incredibly well: the rice, the olives, the feta and a quiet hit of wasabi. Cook the greens over a low heat to keep the crunch and colour. Carrot, Brussels sprouts or fennel tops could also be used for this recipe.

Melt half the butter in a pan, add half the onion and cook gently until soft. Add the rinsed rice and stir until all the grains are coated. Let the rice toast for 1 minute before adding the hot stock a ladleful at a time. Cook the rice as you would risotto, adding the stock gradually, until each addition has been absorbed, stirring frequently, for about 45 minutes, until just tender. Set some of the hot stock aside and stir in wasabi paste to taste.

In another pan, melt the remaining butter, add the remaining onion and cook gently until soft. Add the garlic and continue cooking for a couple of minutes. Add the shredded cima di rapa leaves. Cook over a low heat for a few minutes until tender but still crunchy. Season with salt.

Meanwhile, mix the feta in the chopped olives and oil and leave to marinate. To serve, divide the black rice among serving bowls. Pile on the cima di rapa, then pour over the reserved wasabi stock. Top with the crumbled feta, olives and turnip tops, then serve it on seeded olive crackers.

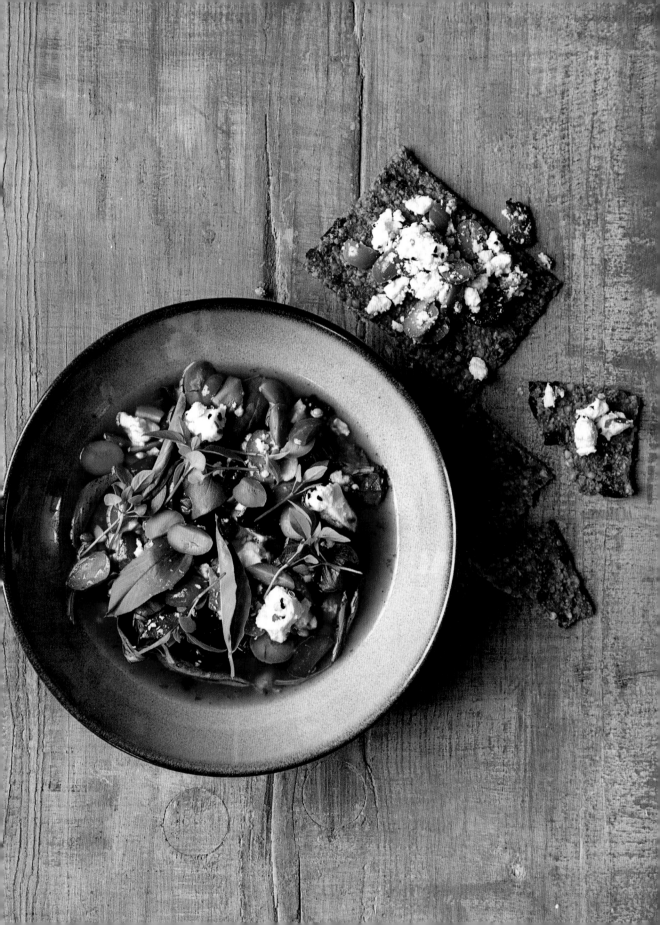

CARROT WITH
TAMARIND & ORANGE

SERVES 4

1 tbsp unsalted butter
800g carrots, roughly chopped
1 litre hot vegetable stock
    (page 15)
1 tbsp tamarind paste
1 orange, zest finely grated
    and juiced
flaky sea salt

We like to buy organic vegetables where possible: the more people support sustainable farming, the more affordable it will become for all of us. Organic carrots don't need to be peeled, unlike ordinary carrots. You just need to give them a bit of a scrub to keep the nutrients found in the skin. A freshly made bowl of carrot soup beats ready-made any day.

Melt the butter in a large saucepan, add the carrots and cook gently for a few minutes. Add the hot vegetable stock to cover, bring to the boil, reduce the heat to a simmer and cook for 20 minutes, or until the carrots are tender. Stir through the tamarind paste, orange zest and juice, season with salt, then process in a blender until smooth. Simple.

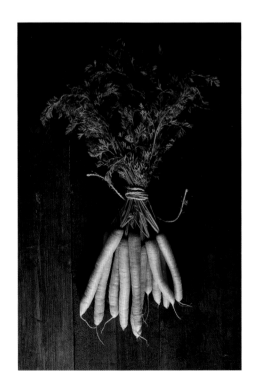

BUTTERNUT SQUASH & CARAMELISED PEAR

SERVES 4

40g unsalted butter
1 onion, finely chopped
1 celery stalk, halved lengthways and finely chopped
1 butternut squash, peeled and cubed
about 1 litre hot vegetable stock (page 15)
2 ripe pears, peeled, cored and cut into 1cm cubes
1 tbsp coconut syrup or sugar
flaky sea salt and freshly ground black pepper

Butternut squash goes with so many things to make delicious, easy soups. It works with chilli, coconut, ginger and cinnamon, or with herbs like rosemary. Here, we've gone for pear and coconut, which are sweet and warming on a chilly day.

Melt half the butter in a heavy-based pan over a low heat, add the onion and cook for 10 minutes, until softened. Add the celery and cook for a few more minutes. Once the onion and celery are translucent, add the butternut squash, then after a minute or so add enough stock to cover the vegetables. Bring to the boil, then reduce the heat to a simmer and cook until the squash is tender, about 10 minutes.

Meanwhile, in a frying pan, melt the remaining butter over a fairly high heat, and once it starts to sizzle, add the pear. Fry for a few minutes, tossing, then add the coconut syrup to the pan and continue frying the pears until golden and caramelised. Process the squash and liquid in a blender, taste and season with salt and pepper, then divide among shallow serving bowls. Add a spoonful of caramelised pear to the centre of each bowl before serving.

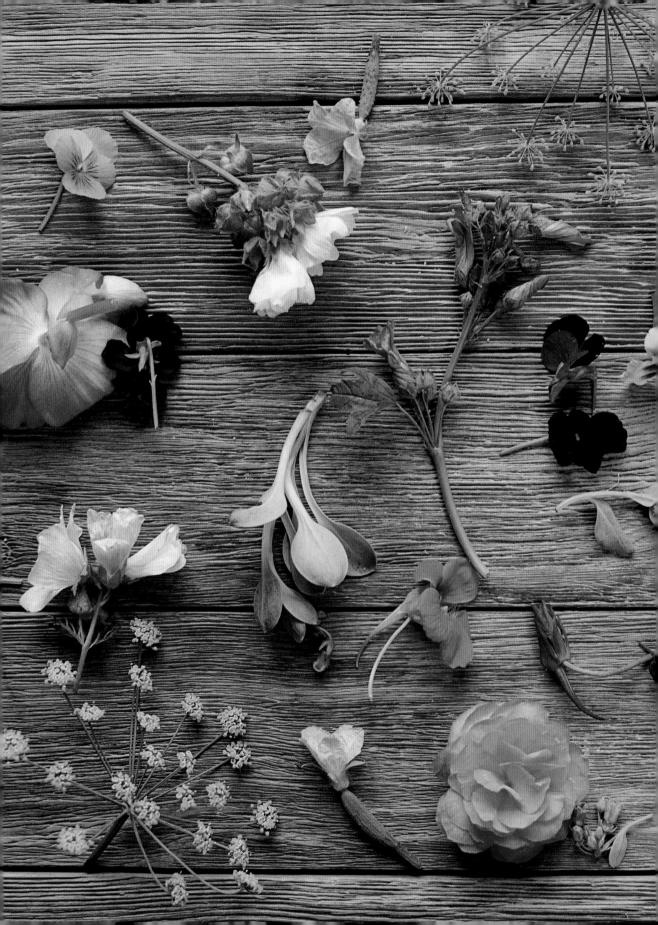

CLEANSING

If you want to change your lifestyle, start with soup

The great thing about soups is that they can give us what we need in so many different ways, whether we crave the restorative heartiness of a beef broth, or just feel an urge to lighten up our diet. Cleansing soups work like juices, but they won't shock your system as much as cold raw foods can. The best cleansing ingredients include nettle, fennel, artichokes (good for the liver), cucumber, green tea, celery and herbs. Yoghurt, along with other fermented foods like pickles, gives us an extra boost of beneficial bacteria, which helps our digestive systems work more efficiently. Soup can also help with weight management: thanks to the water content, it has been shown to be more filling and to keep us fuller for longer compared with eating the same ingredients 'dry'. Of course, soup is packed with nutrients and is usually naturally low in fat,

too. Vegetable soups are an excellent source of soluble fibre, while grains like barley, brown rice and quinoa provide the insoluble type, both of which are helpful for the digestion. If you want to change your lifestyle, start with soup. Eating it instantly makes you feel more healthy, so you'll set up a positive cycle of eating well and have more energy throughout the day.

All in all, soup is the perfect way to clean up your diet and become more adventurous with flavours and ingredients. There are plenty of soups here that need very little preparation, just a well-equipped storecupboard, like our Miso for All Seasons, for example. Lots of the recipes, too, are perfect for whipping up a big batch on the weekend so that you have a super-nutritious meal on hand during the week. What could be easier?

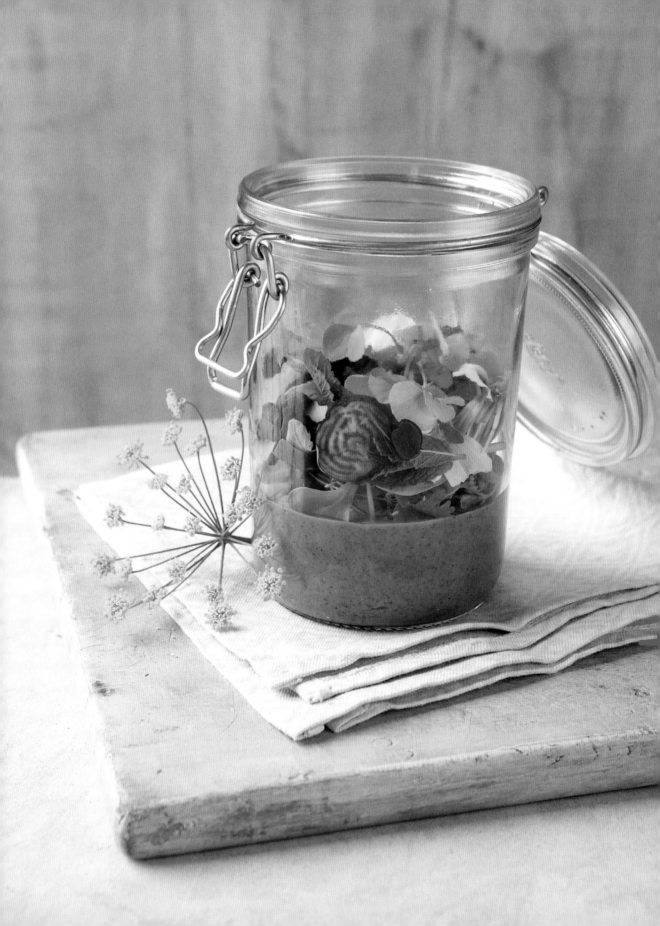

NETTLE SOUP WITH FLOWERS

SERVES 2

1 tbsp olive oil

1½ tbsp unsalted butter

1 banana shallot, finely chopped

1 garlic clove, finely chopped

1 celery stalk, finely chopped

1 bay leaf

a sprig of fresh thyme

200g potatoes, cubed

500ml hot vegetable or
    chicken stock (pages 14–15)

100g nettle tops (about a third
    of a shopping bag's worth of
    pickings)

flaky sea salt

edible flowers (page 71),
    to serve (optional)

Nettles have been used for thousands of years as a tonic, and are now a sought-after ingredient, so let a little wildness into your garden and it will repay you with this lush green soup. Pick just the young, bright green tops of the plants, wearing gloves to avoid stings. Once the leaves hit the hot water their sting will disappear.

Heat the olive oil and half the butter in a heavy-based pan, add the shallot, garlic, celery, bay leaf and thyme, and cook gently for 5–10 minutes, or until soft. Add the potatoes, stir well and continue to cook for a couple of minutes before adding the hot stock.

When the potatoes are tender (about 5–10 minutes), add the nettle tops and cook for 3 minutes, until soft. Remove the bay leaf and thyme, add the remaining butter and process in a blender until smooth. Season with salt and serve with edible flowers if you have them.

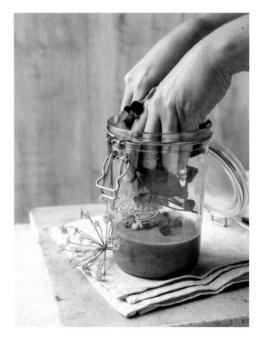

HERB SOUP

SERVES 1

250ml vegetable stock
    (page 15)
1 tbsp white or brown rice,
    rinsed
a bunch of mixed fresh herbs,
    finely chopped, including
    some of the following: mint,
    comfrey, sorrel, borage,
    yarrow, dandelion, basil,
    rosemary, flat-leaf parsley,
    fennel tops, marigold,
    nasturtium leaves or flowers,
    nettles
tamari (soy sauce) or lemon
    juice, to serve (optional)
flaky sea salt and freshly
    ground black pepper

This is the simplest of soups for nourishing body and mind. Spring is traditionally a time to replenish with lots of fresh herbs after the winter months. So if you feel like a new start, take a bunch of herbs and make a pot of soup.

Put the stock and the rice in a small pan, bring to the boil, then reduce the heat and simmer gently until tender (check the instructions on the packet for the cooking time). Taste and season with salt and pepper. Add the freshly chopped herbs and serve immediately. You may like to add either a dash of tamari or lemon juice.

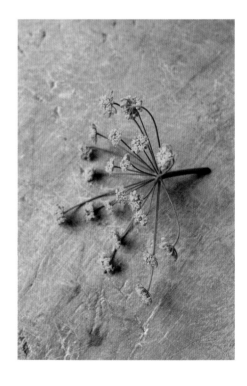

GROW YOUR OWN HERBS

Whether you have a garden, patio, window box or windowsill, growing your own herbs brings wonderful flavours to your cooking in an instant, and it feels good, vibrant and aromatic to have things growing around you. Keep an eye out for unusual edible herbs, too: there are some great mint varieties like chocolate or pineapple mint, and lots of basil varieties to choose from that have spicier flavours. Thyme and rosemary grow well almost anywhere, and have pretty flowers in the spring. These so-called 'woody' herbs are perfect for making bouquet garnis with a couple of bay leaves tied with string. 'Soft' herbs are those such as coriander, dill and basil, which are best chopped and added in the last moments before serving a dish. If you experiment, you'll find out which plants grow best in the soil or light that you have. When preparing a soup or a salad, Nicole will often wait until just before serving to grab a bunch of whatever herb looks and smells good, chop it finely and add to the dish. This never fails to lift all the flavours and give that feeling of freshness.

When it comes to dried herbs, with the exception of rubbed mint, we tend to steer clear of single dried herbs, but we do use them in blends, for example za'atar (page 82), which contains a type of wild thyme that doesn't grow fresh in Europe. The dried seeds, however, do contain some of our favourite flavours, in particular coriander, cumin fennel and mustard seeds.

Edible flowers nourish the heart and might possibly be some of Nicole's favourite things in the world. If you have a garden, you're lucky enough to be able to grow them. Below is a list of some of our favourite herbs along with edible flowers that you can grow from seed, or order as flower 'salads' online (see Resources, page 231).

Soft herbs
Basil
Chervil
Coriander
Chives
Dill
Lemon balm
Lemon verbena
Lovage
Mint
Tarragon
Thai basil

Woody herbs
Bay leaves
Curry leaves
Lemon thyme
Rosemary
Thyme

Edible flowers
Borage flowers
Broad bean flowers
Calendula
Chamomile flowers
Chive flowers
Cornflowers
Courgette flowers
Daisies
Fennel flowers
French marigolds
Lavender
Mallow
Nasturtiums
Radish flowers
Runner bean flowers
Sweet Williams
Violas
Wild garlic flowers

HOT CUCUMBER

SERVES 2

600ml chicken stock (page 14)
1 lemongrass stick, bashed with
    a rolling pin
80g semi-pearled farro, pearl
    barley or spelt
1 small cucumber, peeled,
    de-seeded and sliced
3-4 spring onions, chopped
1 green chilli, thinly sliced
a splash of wheat-free tamari
    (soy) sauce
1 tbsp half-fat crème fraîche
    (optional)
flaky sea salt and freshly
    ground black pepper
fresh root ginger, thinly sliced,
    or pickled ginger, to serve
    (optional)

If you're looking to re-balance after the excesses of the festive season, this soup is full of flavour *and* goodness. It's surprising how good cucumber tastes in a hot soup; it really works! This is one of those soups that you'll urge to cool down a bit so you can eat it more quickly. We use a semi-pearled, quick-cooking variety of farro that only takes 10 minutes to cook. If yours is a wholegrain variety, you'll need to soak it overnight, then cook it for 35–40 minutes.

Bring the chicken stock to the boil in a large pan and reduce the heat to a good simmer. Add the lemongrass and farro. Once the farro is tender (approximately 10 minutes; check the packet instructions, as different types vary), take the pan off the heat and remove the lemongrass. Season to taste.

Add the cucumber, spring onions and chilli and a good splash of tamari sauce. When the soup has cooled a little, stir in the crème fraîche and serve with fresh or pickled ginger on top, if you like.

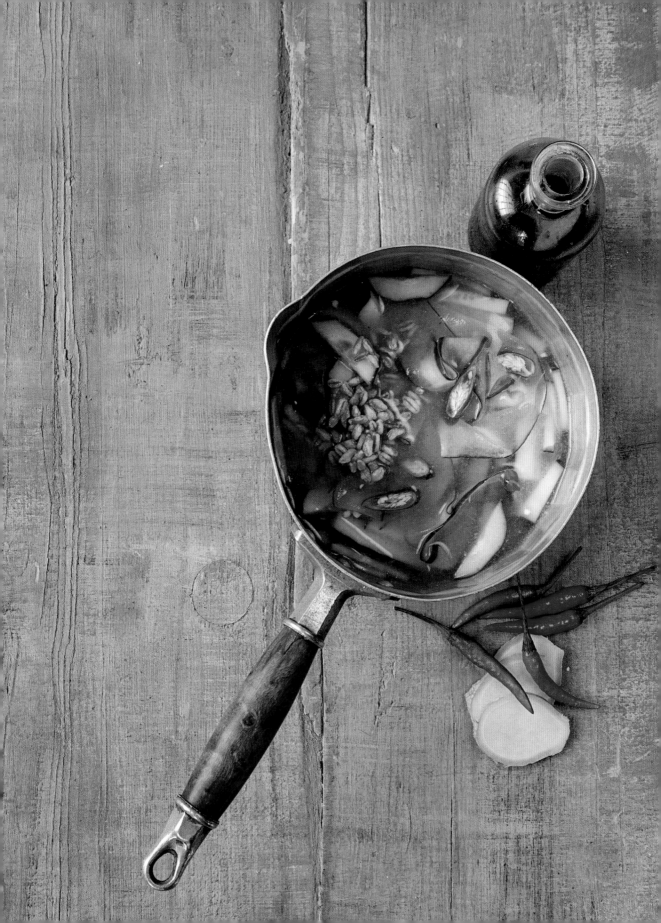

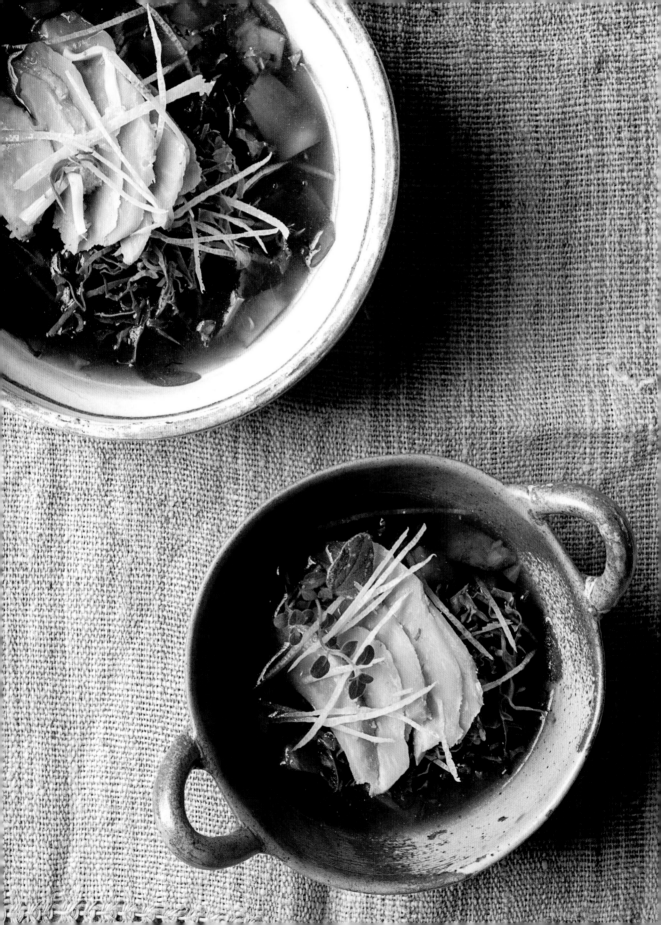

ARTICHOKE BROTH

SERVES 2

4 small artichokes
125ml good-quality white wine
1 tbsp sundried tomato purée
1 tbsp wholegrain mustard
3 tbsp sweet balsamic vinegar
1 tsp ground allspice
1 tsp fennel seeds
¼ tsp flaky sea salt
50g cavolo nero, shredded and
    blanched
zest of 1 unwaxed lemon, cut
    into matchsticks
lemon thyme, to serve
good extra-virgin olive oil,
    to serve

Artichokes are thought to be detoxifying for the liver, helpful for water retention and to ease digestive problems. We've added a little lemon zest to balance out their slightly bitter aftertaste. The small artichokes that arrive in late spring are worth looking out for, and spring is also the best time for our bodies to detox, so it's good for us and the planet to eat with the seasons.

To prepare the artichokes, trim the stems to about 1cm and slice the top 2.5cm off. Snip off the pointy bits of the leaves.

Add 1 litre water to a large pan along with all the other ingredients except the cavolo nero, lemon zest, lemon thyme and extra-virgin olive oil. Bring to the boil, then reduce the heat to a simmer and cook gently for about 1 ½ hours or until the artichokes are tender.

Remove the artichokes and pour the liquid through muslin cloth or a fine sieve, reserving it. Let the artichokes rest. Trim the artichokes by removing the outer leaves until you are left with just the 'hearts' (you can eat the fleshy inner parts of the leaves using a bite and pull technique). Scoop out and discard the inedible fuzzy centres, or chokes, and slice the hearts. Return the hearts to the cooking liquid and warm through. Divide among serving bowls and top with the blanched cavolo nero, lemon zest, lemon thyme and a drizzle of extra-virgin olive oil.

GREEN TEA, BROWN RICE

SERVES 1

75g brown rice, rinsed
250ml hojicha green tea
1 umeboshi plum, chopped
½ tsp furikake seasoning (see
    page 61) or sesame seeds

Tea with rice is a popular snack in Japan, and super-healthy if you're on a bit of a detox. Hojicha is a roasted green tea, and gives a lovely, woody flavour (see Resources, page 231). You could also use sencha green tea, which is more widely available and has a fresher taste. Umeboshi plums (see page 231) have a surprising flavour, a hint of sweet with quite a strong saltiness. As an alternative you could top the soup with hot smoked salmon, trout or mackerel, and add pickled ginger or some cooked beetroot.

Cook the brown rice in boiling water according to the instructions on the packet. Meanwhile, make a pot of hojicha green tea; the trick is not to use just-boiled water, which will burn the tea, but wait a minute until the water cools slightly before pouring it over the leaves. Brew for about 7 minutes (a perfect amount of time for calming the mind). Put the rice in a serving bowl, pour over the tea and garnish with the plum and furikake seasoning.

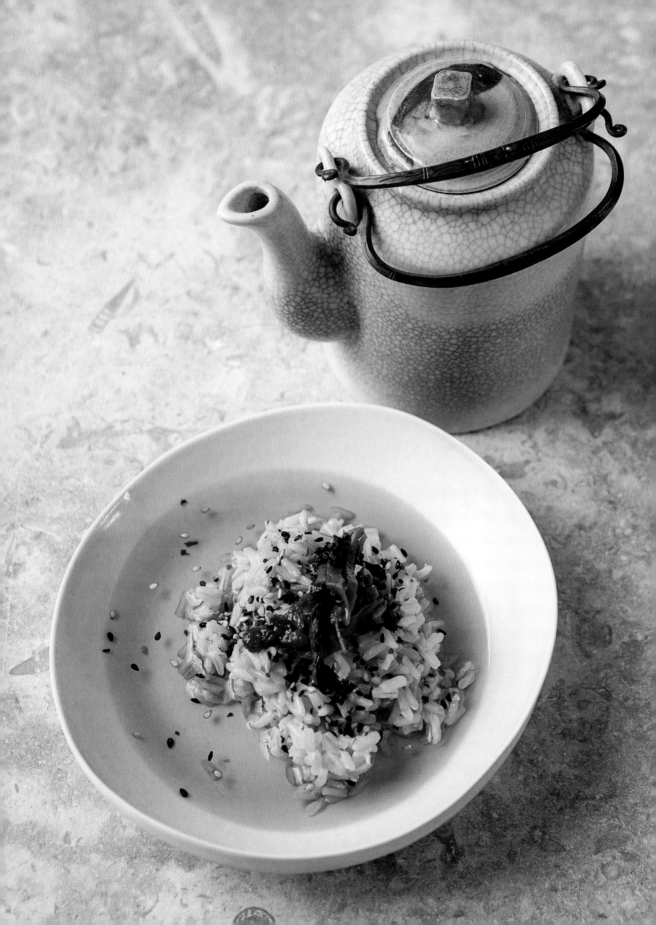

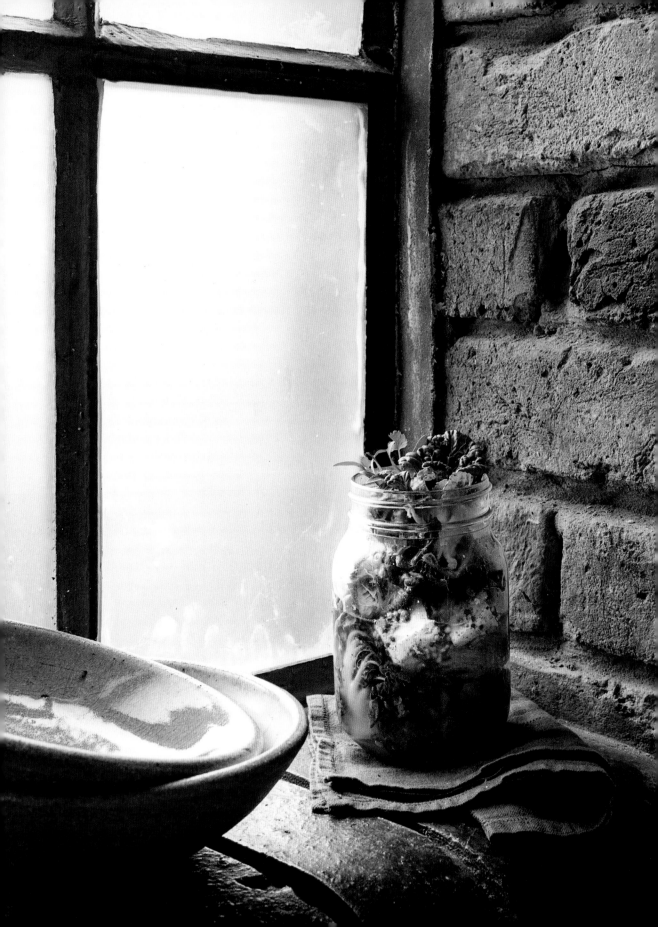

FIVE-SPICE & THREE-LEAF

SERVES 2

200g firm, fresh tofu, drained
  and cut into 2cm cubes
½ tsp mustard seeds, crushed
½ tsp fennel seeds, crushed
½ tsp black onion seeds,
  crushed
½ tsp flaky sea salt
½ tsp ground Chinese five-spice
  (cinnamon, fennel, star anise,
  ginger, cloves)
1 tsp white miso paste
unsalted butter, for frying
100g mixed leafy greens such
  as bok choy, swiss chard, tat
  soi or cabbage, sliced finely

The beauty of tofu is that it takes on so many flavours. Although you might have been put off it in the past if all you've eaten is tasteless, rubbery tofu that no one in their right minds would enjoy, give it a chance in this dish. The spiced tofu is a brilliant stand-by for a variety of instant, healthy lunches, for example with hummus and avocado or a big bunch of wilted baby spinach.

Put the tofu cubes in a bowl with the mustard seeds, fennel seeds, black onion seeds, salt and Chinese five-spice and toss to coat. You can use it immediately or leave it to marinate in the refrigerator until you need it (it will keep well for 3 days).

Dissolve the white miso paste in 400ml boiling water. Melt the butter in a frying pan, add the greens and sauté gently for 2–3 minutes, until tender. Layer the greens and tofu in serving bowls or large glass Kilner jars and add white miso broth to serve.

MISO FOR ALL SEASONS

SPRING MISO FOR ONE
1 white miso soup sachet
1 small baby gem lettuce,
    shredded
a small handful of fresh
    petit pois
alfalfa sprouts, to garnish

SUMMER MISO FOR ONE
a large handful of kale,
    shredded
1 tbsp light olive oil
1 tbsp pumpkin seeds
a small handful of green beans,
    sliced lengthways
1 red miso soup sachet
flaky sea salt

AUTUMN MISO FOR ONE
1 brown miso soup sachet
a small handful of enoki
    mushrooms
1 tsp unsalted butter
1 egg yolk

WINTER MISO FOR ONE
1 white miso soup sachet
a handful of watercress leaves
a small handful of radish, very
    thinly sliced

Miso soup sachets are the new cup-a-soups, and they happen to be packed with goodness, too. Miso soup is served as an accompaniment to Japanese meals, but we decided to make more of a meal out of it and experiment with some seasonal additions. Now we have no excuse for not being able to start a health kick any time of the year! You can find miso soup sachets in most supermarkets and all health-food shops.

SPRING MISO FOR ONE
Prepare the soup according to the instructions on the packet, add the lettuce and petit pois and garnish with alfalfa sprouts just before serving.

SUMMER MISO FOR ONE
Preheat the oven to 140°C/fan 120°C/275°F/gas mark 1. Toss the shredded kale in light olive oil and a good pinch of salt. Spread it out on an oven tray and bake for about 20 minutes, turning it halfway through, until crispy. Add the pumpkin seeds for the last 5 minutes. This also makes a brilliant snack on its own. Boil the green beans in water for a couple of minutes, until just tender.

Prepare the soup according to the instructions on the packet and add the crispy kale, green beans and pumpkin seeds.

AUTUMN MISO FOR ONE
Prepare the soup according to the instructions on the packet. Fry the enoki mushrooms in a little butter and poach the egg yolk by bringing a small saucepan of water to a simmer, gently lowering the yolk into the water and poaching for 1–2 minutes, until just set. Add the mushrooms to the soup and top with the poached yolk.

WINTER MISO FOR ONE
Prepare the soup according to the instructions on the packet, add the watercress and radishes then serve.

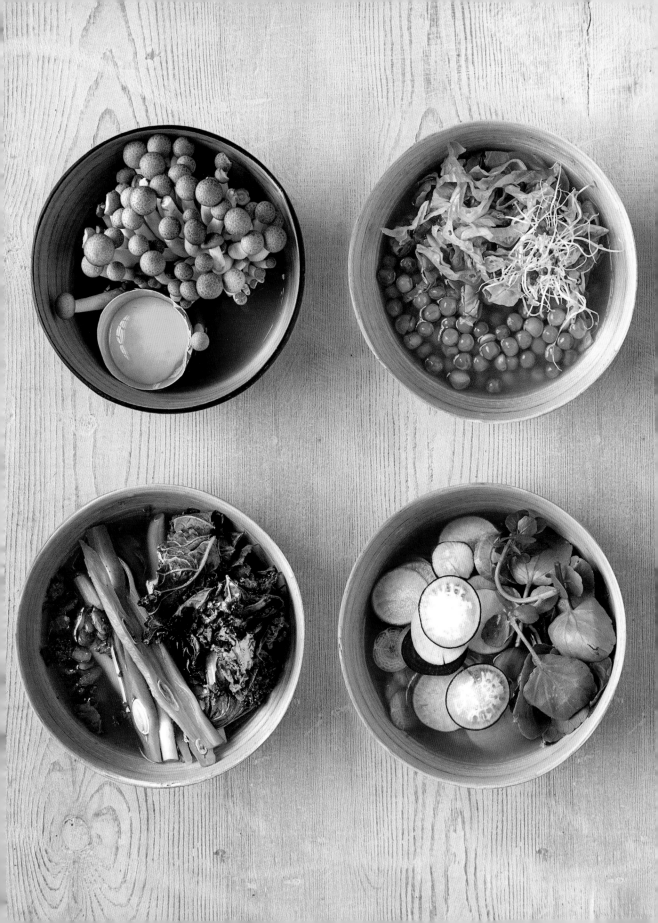

LOVE YOUR
SPICE CUPBOARD

Spices are one of the simplest and healthiest ways to expand your cooking repertoire, so show your spice cupboard some love! Collect all your spices together and throw out any that are beyond their use-by date. Arrange them so that you can actually see them, otherwise it's so easy to forget what you have and use the same ones again and again. Plan a dinner around your spice cupboard by exploring your cookbooks for new ways to use spices.

Spices often have health benefits, too. In particular, warming spices such as ginger, cinnamon, cumin, nutmeg and coriander aid digestion. And turmeric, which is in the same family as ginger, is one of the healthiest foods available; it may be helpful for arthritis, maintaining weight, reducing cholesterol, healing wounds, relieving eczema and candida and protecting the liver. We've included a comprehensive list of the everyday spices you'll need on page 11. Here are some less well-known favourite spices and blends that are also well worth seeking out. Turn to the resources listed on page 231 for some great spice stockists.

Dukkah: A blend of spices, often made with hazelnuts, sesame seeds, coriander, cumin and paprika.

Za'atar: A herb that grows in the Syrian-Lebanese mountains, sometimes called wild thyme in English, since it has a thyme-like flavour. Za'atar is also the name of a spice blend, often made with wild thyme, olive oil, toasted sesame seeds and sumac.

Ras el hanout: This North African spice mix is often used in Moroccan cooking. The name literally translates as 'top of the shop', which probably derives from the fact that it is traditionally made with the best spices available, including cardamom, cloves, cinnamon, rose buds and lavender.

Baharat: A warming Middle Eastern spice blend that contains black pepper, cumin, coriander, cinnamon, cloves, cardamom, nutmeg and paprika.

Urfa chilli flakes: These pepper flakes have a wonderful, smoky, slightly sweet flavour that adds a little heat without overpowering.

Grains of paradise: These West African seeds are similar to black pepper, but more subtle, and we can't resist the name.

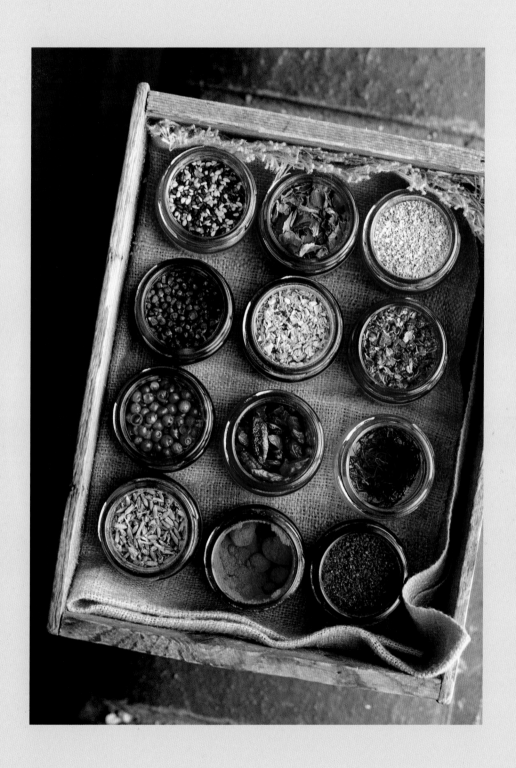

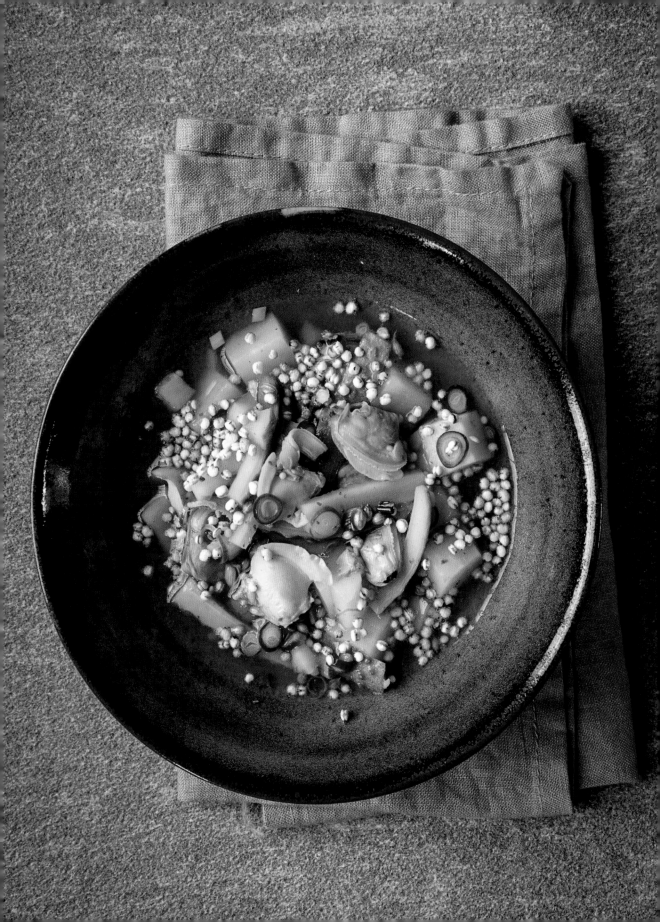

PICKLED SOUP

SERVES 2

½ tbsp unsalted butter
½ onion, chopped
200g new potatoes, preferably
    Jersey Royal, cubed
½ tsp ground or 1 tsp grated
    fresh turmeric
400ml hot seaweed and
    mushroom or vegetable
    stock (pages 17 and 15)
6 lily bulb flakes or 1 garlic
    clove, thinly sliced
2 tbsp puffed quinoa or
    toasted pine nuts

For the pickled cucumber
2 small cucumbers, sliced
200ml apple cider vinegar
6 cardamom pods
½ tsp ground or 1 tsp grated
    fresh turmeric
100g raw cane sugar

For the pickled clams
500g fresh clams in their shells
50ml cider
200ml apple cider vinegar
1 tbsp pink peppercorns

We came across lily bulbs in our local Asian store and discovered that you can use them as you would use a herb, in a soup or stir-fry for example. They are traditionally used as a remedy for coughs and colds, which makes sense as they do look quite similar to garlic, which you could happily use instead. We also happened to have some pickled cucumber and clams in the fridge, and Nicole rustled up a very tasty pickled soup.

For the pickled cucumber, put the cucumber slices into a sterilised preserving jar, packing them in snugly. Heat the remaining ingredients for the cucumber in a pan with 400ml water, bring just to the boil and simmer for 3-4 minutes. Pour the hot liquid carefully over the cucumber slices, fasten the lid and allow to sit for about 1 hour before putting in the fridge. Once sealed, they should keep for up to a month.

For the pickled clams, rinse the clams thoroughly and discard any that remain open. Heat a large pan and once hot add the clams. Add the cider and cover with a lid, then simmer until the shells have opened (discard any clams that remain closed). Strain the clams, reserving the cooking liquid, and remove the clams from the shells. Pack them into a small sterilised preserving jar. Heat the cooking liquid with the apple cider vinegar and pink peppercorns. When hot, pour enough of the liquid over the clams to cover, seal the jar and allow to sit for about 1 hour before putting in the fridge.

To make the soup, melt the butter in a saucepan, add the onion and cook gently until soft. Add the potatoes and turmeric and cook, stirring, for 1 minute before adding the hot stock and lily bulb flakes. Bring to the boil and simmer until the potatoes are cooked, about 15-20 minutes. Add a quarter of the pickled cucumber and 4 tablespoons pickled clams just to warm them through before serving in deep bowls. Sprinkle with puffed quinoa to serve.

CELERY SOUP WITH BEETROOT-CURED SALMON

SERVES 2

50g unsalted butter
400g celery, finely chopped
1 onion, finely chopped
1 potato (about 200g), diced
800ml chicken or vegetable
    stock (pages 14–15)
2 tsp finely chopped fresh dill,
    plus extra to garnish
flaky sea salt and freshly
    ground white pepper
fromage frais, to serve

For the cured salmon
500g boneless salmon fillet in
    one piece, skin on
300g cooked beetroot
300g smoked flaky sea salt
300g coconut sugar or raw
    cane sugar

When Nicole talks about 'clean' food what she really means is that the food is simple, not fussy, and that the combined tastes work well together. The flavours of this soup are indeed simple and, yes, clean: celery, salmon, dill and a hint of beetroot.

To make the cured salmon, remove any remaining pin bones with tweezers or the tip of a knife. Process the beetroot in a blender or food processor to make a paste, add the salt and sugar and put half the mixture in a shallow dish that is the same size as the salmon. Place the salmon on top, skin-side down, then cover with another layer of beetroot mixture so that the salmon is completely covered. Allow to cure for 24 hours in the refrigerator. Remove the salmon from the cure, gently rinse it, pat dry with kitchen paper and then thinly slice it.

To make the soup, melt the butter in a heavy-based pan over a low heat and add the celery, onion and potato. Cover with a lid and cook gently for 10 minutes, stirring occasionally, without allowing it to colour. Add the stock and half the dill, bring to the boil, then reduce the heat to a simmer and cook gently for another 15–20 minutes, or until the vegetables are tender. Process the soup in batches in a blender, then push it through a sieve into a clean saucepan to remove any celery strings. Taste and season with salt and pepper. Divide the soup among serving bowls and garnish with the remaining dill and slivers of cured salmon, with fromage frais on the side.

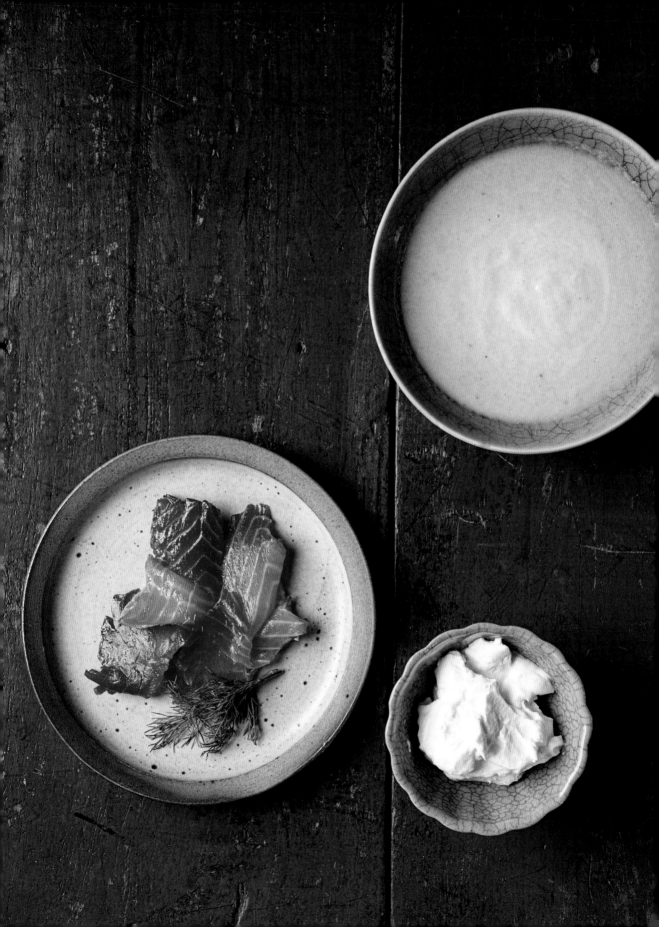

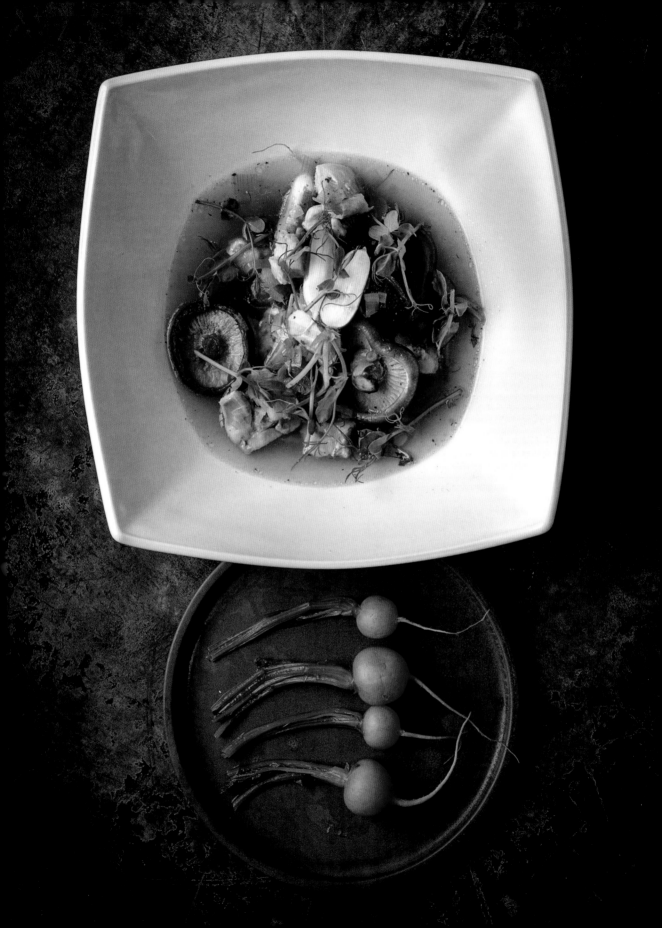

HAPPY NEW YEAR OZONI

SERVES 4

1 litre seaweed and mushroom
   stock (page 17)
200g skinless chicken thigh
   fillets, cut into bite-sized
   pieces
1 small leek, sliced on an angle
   1.5cm thick
4 fresh shiitake mushrooms,
   with crosses cut into the
   centres
50g daikon or white turnip
1½ tbsp tamari (soy) sauce
2 tbsp white miso paste
12 French Breakfast radishes,
   halved lengthways
flaky sea salt
unwaxed lemon zest, grated,
   to serve
pea shoots, to serve

Traditionally, this classic Japaneses soup is made on New Year's Eve. What a perfect, healthy way to make a fresh start to the year! We fell in love with the book *Zenbu Zen* by Jane Lawson. It describes Jane's experiences of discovering 'food, culture and balance' in Kyoto, and it's both beautiful and mouthwatering. We've adapted her ozoni soup here.

Daikon are very large, mildly flavoured radishes and you will only need a few slices for this soup. Use the leftover daikon in a coleslaw, try it roasted or add it to stews.

Bring the stock to the boil in a large saucepan. Add the chicken, leek, mushrooms and daikon and simmer, skimming off any foamy residue from the surface. Cook for 15 minutes, or until the daikon is just starting to soften.

Mix together the tamari sauce and miso paste. Add a little of the hot cooking liquid to dissolve the miso, then pour it into the pan along with the radishes and stir to combine. Season the soup with salt to taste. Ladle the broth into 4 serving bowls. Sprinkle with lemon zest and pea shoots, then serve immediately.

YOGHURT SOUP

SERVES 1

white wine vinegar, for
poaching the eggs
2 eggs
150g natural yoghurt
1 tbsp chilli oil
flaky sea salt
wood sorrel, to garnish
(optional)
slices of toasted ciabatta,
to serve

Breakfast is one of our favourite things in the world, so here's a soup you could really call brunch. Use the freshest eggs you can find to help make the perfect poached eggs.

Preheat the oven to 140°C/fan 120°C/285°F/gas mark 1.

Bring a saucepan of water to the boil and add a small splash of white vinegar. Crack each egg into an individual ramekin or small bowl. Create a 'whirlpool' effect in the water by stirring it vigorously in one direction. Gently tip each egg from its ramekin into the middle of the water. Poach for 3 minutes, then remove with a slotted spoon and drain on kitchen paper.

Meanwhile warm the yoghurt by pouring it into an ovenproof dish and placing it in the oven for 5 minutes.

Put the yoghurt in a serving bowl and top it with the poached eggs. Add a drizzle of chilli oil, garnish with wood sorrel (if using) and sprinkle over some sea salt. Serve with toasted ciabatta to dip into the eggs and yoghurt.

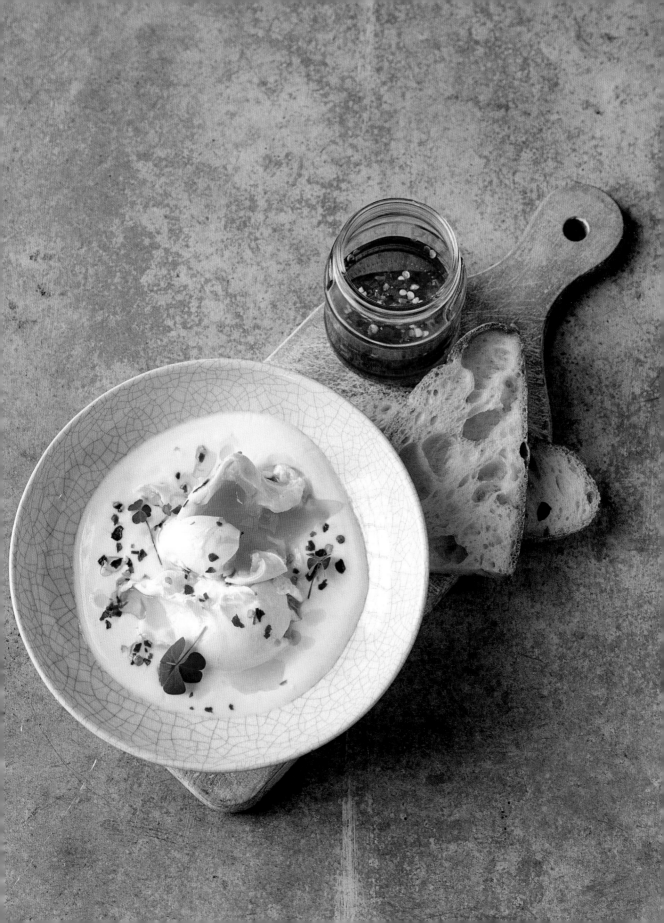

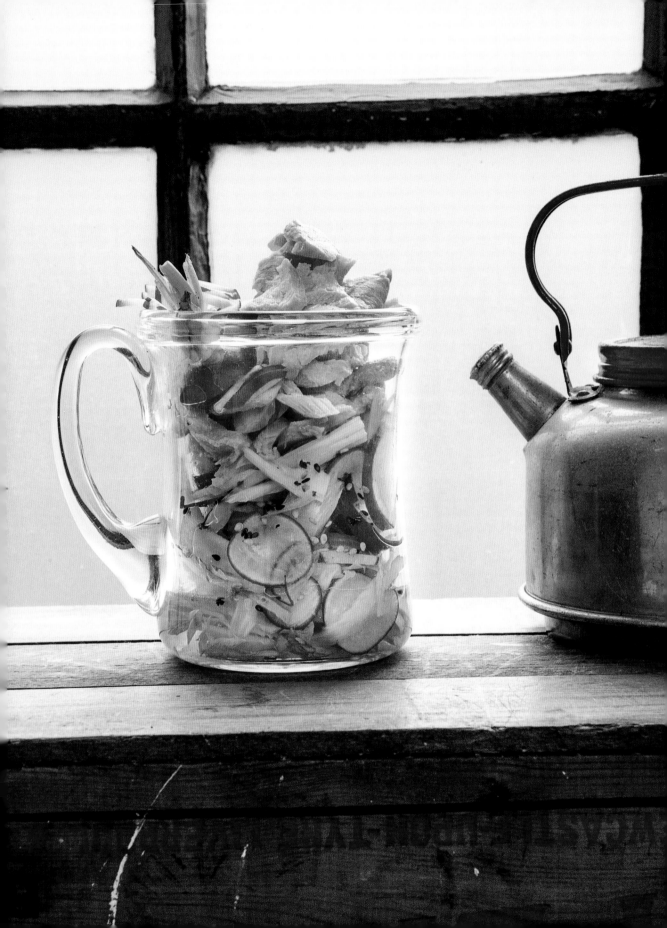

SALMON POACHED IN LEMONGRASS TEA

SERVES 2

a large pot of freshly brewed
   lemongrass tea (about 1 litre)
1 salmon fillet, approximately 150g
1 celery stalk, sliced lengthways
a small handful of radishes,
   thinly sliced
furikake seasoning, optional
   (see page 61)
flaky sea salt and freshly
   ground black pepper

Nicole has never had a taste for drinking herbal tea in the conventional way. So, being a chef, she came up with a recipe using it instead.

Bring the tea halfway up to the boil in a pan and add the salmon fillet. Poach for about 8 minutes, or until the flesh is just nicely flaking. Remove the salmon and flake the flesh, discarding the skin.

Divide the celery and radish among the serving bowls. Add the salmon flakes, then pour over the remaining hot tea. Season with furikake (if using), salt and pepper, then serve.

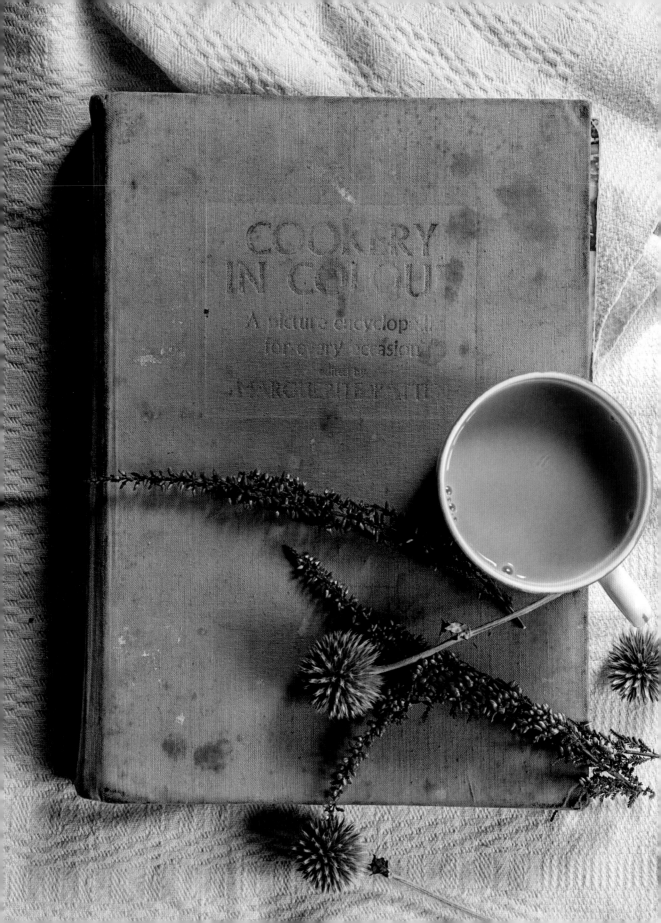

OLD WIVES' TALES

'Worries go down better with
soup than without.'

JEWISH PROVERB

Many people believe that old remedies and healing soups from traditional health philosophies such as Chinese medicine or Ayurveda can help us listen to and understand our bodies. Drawing on many centuries of experience, cultures around the world have developed bone broths or rice-based soups that help us recuperate and recover, and chicken soup recipes have been passed down through the generations along with secret ingredients and tall tales.

The story of the recipe for Stone Soup is a good example: one day, a weary traveller arrived at the edge of a village in the Swiss countryside. He noticed a kind-looking woman sitting in her doorway. Eventually, after they had talked for a while, the traveller asked the woman if she had a fire, to which she replied that of course she did, how else could she cook her family's dinner? The pot was already warming water over the fire. The man asked if she would be so good as to lend

him some of the warm water. She was curious about why he wanted it, to which he said, 'Oh, well, if you might also lend me your pot, I can show you.' So the woman lent him her pot and asked him what he was going to make. The man told her he would make Stone Soup, and produced a large, smooth pebble from his pocket. He explained that the stone was the main ingredient, but if she could provide him with some bread, a bit of meat and a few vegetables, he would have everything he needed. She kindly gave him the ingredients she had to hand in her garden and kitchen cupboards, as well as a few herbs. After some time, he finished making the soup and they shared it together. As a thank you, the traveller gave the woman the stone and told her if she always made soup with it just as they had that day it would always taste as good. She revealed the discovery to her neighbours, who passed it on again, and so Stone Soup was etched into folklore.

APPLE CIDER BEETROOT

SERVES 2

4 large or 6 small whole
    beetroot
2 tbsp apple cider vinegar
300-400ml hot chicken or
    vegetable stock (pages
    14-15), depending on how
    thick you like your soup
2 tbsp chopped fresh dill
sour cream, to serve
dried edible rose petals,
    to garnish (optional)
flaky sea salt

Cider vinegar has been used in home remedies for thousands
of years, and it is thought that Hippocrates (the godfather of
medicine) used it as an elixir. You can find all kinds of vinegars these
days, from raspberry to pomegranate, but for pickling, good old
cider vinegar is still one of the best. Here the beetroot is roasted,
keeping its wonderful colour and flavour. This soup is simple to
prepare and gives a delicious result every time.

Preheat the oven to 200°C/fan 180°C/400°F/gas mark 6. Wash the
beetroot and cut off all but 2.5cm of the stalks. Place in a roasting
tray and add enough water to come about halfway up the sides, plus
the vinegar. Cover with foil and bake for 40-45 minutes, or until soft.

Allow the beetroot to cool, and then rub off the skins with kitchen
paper. Roughly chop the beetroot, then blend with the stock and
chopped dill. Season with salt. Serve warm or cold with sour cream
and a few rose petals if you like.

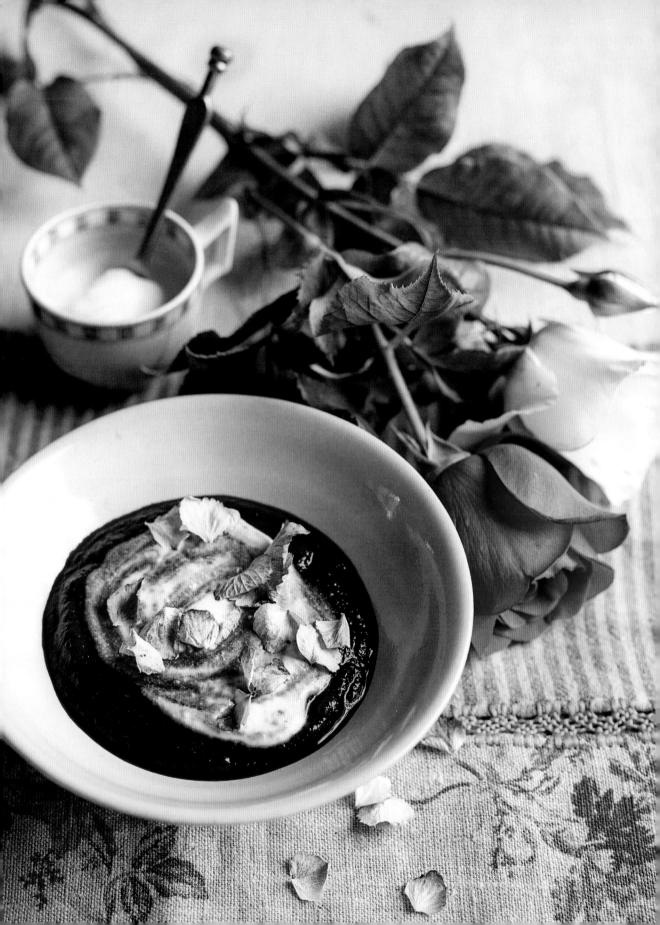

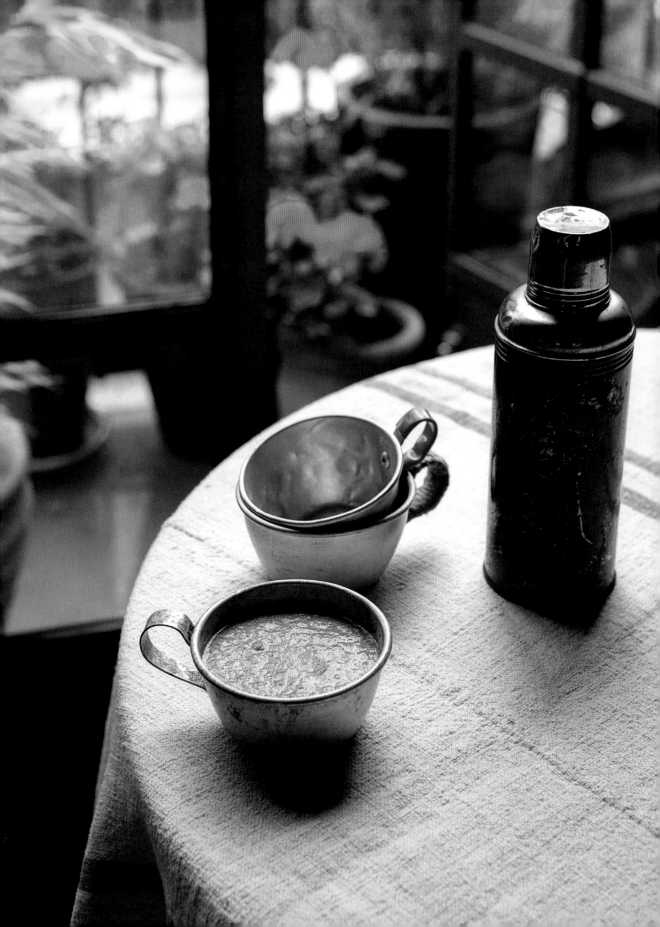

GOOD WOMAN'S SOUP

SERVES 4

100g lovage leaves
20g unsalted butter
1 onion, sliced
1 cos lettuce, chopped
400g peas (fresh or frozen)
1 tbsp fresh tarragon or chervil,
    chopped, plus extra to serve
800ml hot chicken or
    vegetable stock (pages 14–15)
4 slices ciabatta bread
2 tbsp olive oil
1 tbsp balsamic vinegar
flaky sea salt and freshly
    ground black pepper

This is adapted from a soup recipe we found in *Mrs Beeton's Book of Household Management*. We couldn't resist the name! It's very good on a hot summer day when you're bored of salad.

Bring a pan of water to the boil and blanch the lovage leaves for a few seconds. Drain under cold water and place on a clean kitchen towel, squeezing out any excess moisture.

Melt the butter in a large heavy-based pan, add the onion and cook gently until softened. After about 10 minutes, add the lettuce, peas and tarragon and give everything a good stir for 1 minute before adding the hot stock. Once the peas are cooked – about 4 minutes – process in a blender until smooth. Taste and season with salt and pepper.

To make croutons, cut the ciabatta slices into small cubes. Heat the olive oil in a pan and fry the cubes, adding the balsamic vinegar until crisp. Serve the hot soup immediately, topped with croutons and freshly chopped tarragon, or to serve cold you might prefer to pass it through a sieve for a thinner soup before refrigerating.

MAGIC SOUP

SERVES 2

250g yellow split peas
1/4 tsp cayenne pepper
1/2 tsp ground turmeric
1 tbsp coconut oil or unsalted
    butter
1 onion, sliced
1/2 tsp cinnamon
1/2 tsp ground ginger
1/2 tsp garam masala (or a
    mixture of cumin, black
    pepper, nutmeg, cardamom,
    cassia, cloves)
180g young leaf spinach
2 tbsp toasted mixed seeds
    (such as sunflower seeds,
    pumpkin seeds or sesame
    seeds)

Magic soup, Kate discovered, is what Mauritian women eat after having a baby to get back in shape while getting as much nutrition as possible. We fell in love with the name and it always reminds us to make a batch of soup when we're feeling in need of a burst of delicious healthiness. We've created a version of our own, with a combination of the best metabolism-boosting, fat-burning spices, including cayenne pepper, turmeric, cinnamon, ginger, black pepper, cardamom and cumin.

Rinse the split peas thoroughly and put them in a saucepan with 1 litre water, the cayenne pepper and turmeric, and bring to the boil. Reduce the heat to a simmer and cook gently for about 50 minutes, or until the split peas are soft and broken up. Remove half the split peas and process to a smooth consistency in a blender (or use a stick blender), then return them to the pan with the rest and stir through.

Heat the coconut oil in a large frying pan, add the onion and cook gently for about 10 minutes, or until soft. Add the spices and continue to cook for about 5 minutes, until the aromas are released. Add the spinach to the pan and stir until it has wilted. Heat through the split pea soup, divide among 2 serving bowls and top with the spiced spinach and onions. Garnish with toasted mixed seeds.

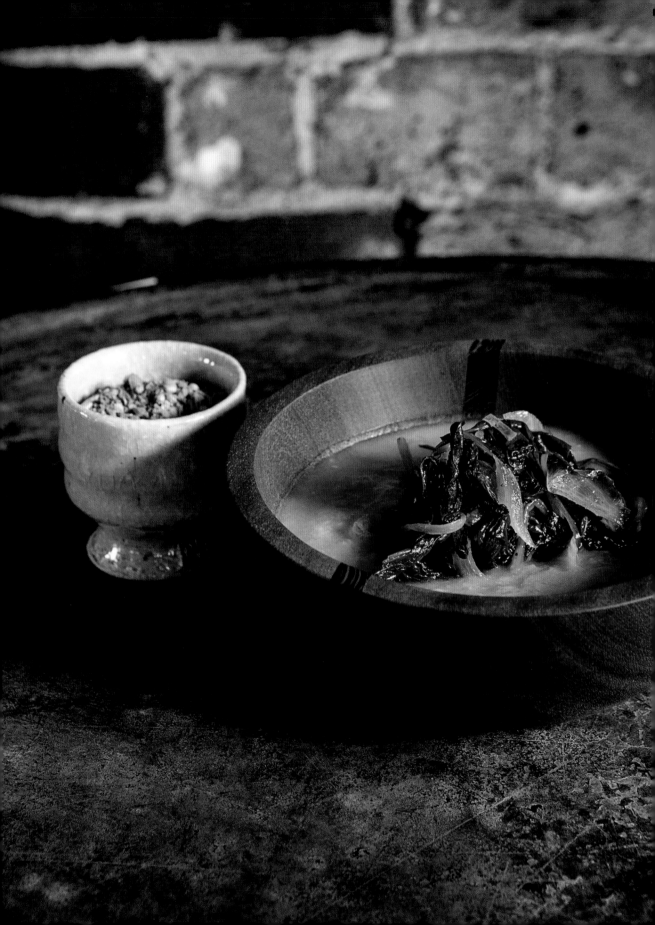

CABBAGE SOUP
REINVENTED

SERVES 4-6

olive oil, for frying

2 leek and apple sausages,
   sliced

1 onion, finely diced

1 carrot, finely diced

1 celery stalk, finely diced

500g green lentils, rinsed

1 bay leaf

a sprig of fresh thyme or
   rosemary

1-1.2 litres hot chicken stock
   (page 14), depending on how
   thick you like your soup

1 Savoy cabbage, outer leaves
   removed, and very finely
   shredded

flaky sea salt and freshly
   ground black pepper

Nobody knows for sure where the cabbage soup diet originated, but if you were to eat cabbage soup all day for a couple of weeks, you're sure to lose a few pounds (along with a few friends). Cabbage soup can, however, be delicious, with the addition of sausages. These can go a really long way in a soup, so you can have a bit of what you fancy.

Heat a little oil in a large saucepan and fry the sausage pieces until cooked through. Remove and set aside. Add the onion, carrot and celery to the pan and sweat gently for about 15 minutes.

Return the sausages to the pan, along with the lentils, and give everything a good stir. Add the bay leaf and thyme, and then the hot stock. Bring to the boil, reduce the heat to a simmer and cook for 25-30 minutes (check the instructions on the lentil packet). Stir in the shredded cabbage 5 minutes before the lentils are cooked through. Season with salt and pepper.

BONE BROTHS
& HOSPITAL DIETS

When Nicole is feeling poorly she'll make Bovril pasta, which is a modern equivalent of the bone broths that have been used for centuries to strengthen the weak. The first restaurants in Paris served *restauratifs* (restoratives), in other words, bone broths; and in Chinese medicine, which is thousands of years old, chicken soup is highly revered as a healing soup, since it contains the essence of the marrow. Beef or chicken broth may take a little patience, but the depth of flavour obtained is worth letting a pot simmer for a few hours. The early English food writer Hannah Glasse, who wrote cookery books for household staff, gave a number of convalescence recipes, including these two soups.

Beef-Drink, which is ordered for weak People

Take a pound of lean beef, then take off all the fat and skin, cut it into pieces, put it into a gallon of water, with the under-crust of a penny-loaf, and a very little salt. Let it boil till it comes to two quarts, then strain it off, and it is a very hearty drink.

Bread Soup for the Sick

Take a quart of water, set it on the fire in a clean saucepan, and as much dry crust of bread cut to pieces as the top of a penny-loaf, the drier the better, a bit of butter as big as a walnut; let it boil, then beat it with a spoon, and keep boiling it till the bread and water is well mixed; then season it with very little salt, and it is a pretty thing for a weak stomach.

From *The Art of Cookery Made Plain and Easy* (1747)

Alexis Soyer was a French chef who gave an account of his time at the front in the Crimean War, which included recipes for the injured soldiers, the 'hospital diet'.

Semi-stewed Mutton and Barley Soup

Mutton joint, mixed vegetables, barley, salt, flour, sugar, pepper

Put all the ingredients into the pan at once, except the flour; set it on the fire, and when beginning to boil, diminish the heat, and simmer gently for 2 hours and a half; take the joint(s) of meat out, and keep them warm in the orderly's pan; add to the soup your flour, which you have mixed with enough water to form a light batter; stir well together with a large spoon; boil another half-hour, skim off the fat, and serve the soup and meat separate. The meat may be put back into the soup for a few minutes to warm again prior to serving. The soup should be stirred now and then while making, to prevent burning or sticking to the bottom of the caldron.

The joints are cooked whole, and afterwards cut up … being cooked this way, in a rather thick stock, the meat becomes more nutritious.

From *A Culinary Campaign* (1857)

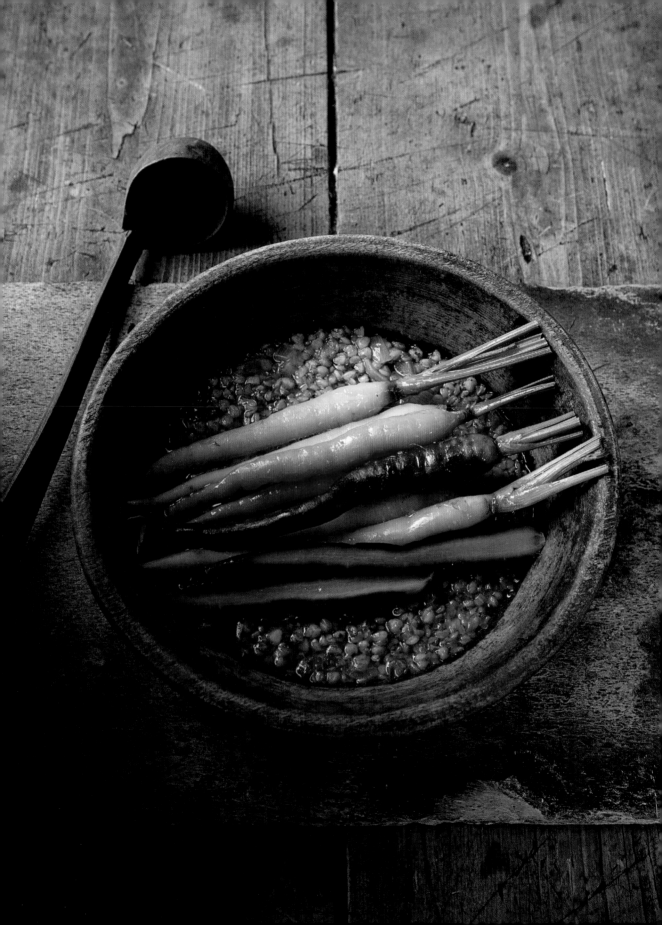

CARROT & ROASTED BUCKWHEAT

SERVES 4

1 tbsp coconut oil

1 onion, finely chopped

2 celery stalks, finely chopped

2 tsp grated fresh root ginger

2 garlic cloves, crushed

150g roasted buckwheat

1.2 litres hot chicken or
   vegetable stock (pages 14–15)

400g baby carrots or heritage
   carrots, washed and
   scrubbed

zest of ½ orange

zest of ½ lemon

knob unsalted butter

flaky sea salt and freshly
   ground black pepper

This is the perfect winter detox soup: it's warming, comforting and good for you. The carrots and ginger help your digestive system, as does the roasted buckwheat, which has a delicious nutty flavour. Despite the name, it's actually a fruit seed, so it's an excellent gluten-free alternative if you struggle with grains. You can find it in health-food shops, Polish shops and online.

Heat the coconut oil in a heavy-based pan and add the onion and celery. Cover with a lid and cook gently over a low heat for 10 minutes. Add the ginger and garlic and give everything a good stir for about 1 minute before adding the roasted buckwheat and 1 litre of the hot stock. Bring to the boil, then reduce the heat to a simmer and cook gently for another 15 minutes. Taste and season with salt and pepper.

Meanwhile, heat the remaining stock in a separate pan and braise the baby carrots gently until tender – about 10 minutes, depending on their size. Toss the carrots with the citrus zest along with the butter. To serve, ladle the buckwheat broth into shallow bowls and top with the baby carrots.

COLIN'S CULLEN SKINK

SERVES 2–3

325g potatoes, diced
1 tsp coconut oil
1 tsp unsalted butter
4 leeks, trimmed (green parts
    reserved), diced
570ml whole milk
280g (2 fillets) undyed smoked
    haddock
flaky sea salt and freshly
    ground black pepper

Our friend Colin is from Glasgow, and since the Scottish seem to make and consume more soup than just about any other country in the world, we had to ask him for his favourite one. It's named after the town of Cullen in Moray, and is perfect after a long walk in the Highlands.

Bring a pan of salted water to the boil, add the potatoes and cook until tender, then drain well. Meanwhile, melt the oil and butter in a large frying pan, add the white parts of the leeks and fry gently until soft. Remove and set aside. Add the milk to the same pan with the haddock and the green parts of the leeks. The haddock should be just covered by the milk. Bring to the boil, reduce the heat to a simmer and cook gently for 4 minutes, then cover, remove from the heat and leave to stand for 5 minutes.

Process the fried leeks to a purée in a food processor, adding a spoonful of milk from the haddock pan if needed. Mash the cooked potatoes and divide them into 2 equal quantities. Add the blitzed leeks to half the potatoes.

Remove the haddock from the pan and check that it is cooked through but still retains a very slight bit of translucency in the centre. Strain the milk from the pan and add the cooking liquid to the leek and potato mixture to make the base of the soup.

Process one of the haddock fillets until smooth in a food processor, then add it to the leek and potato soup base. Flake the second haddock fillet into the soup. Finally, stir in the reserved mashed potatoes and serve.

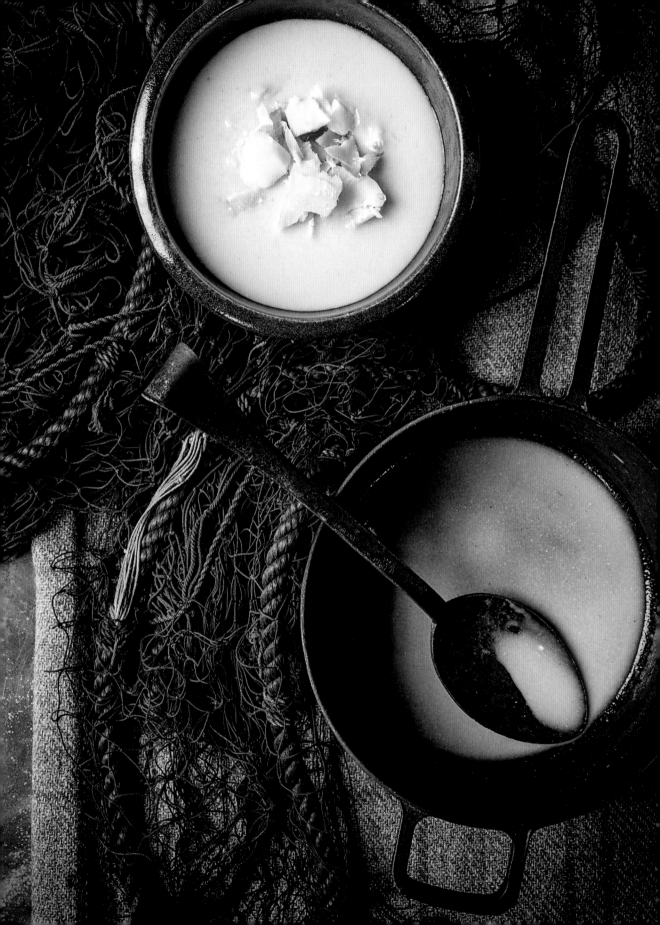

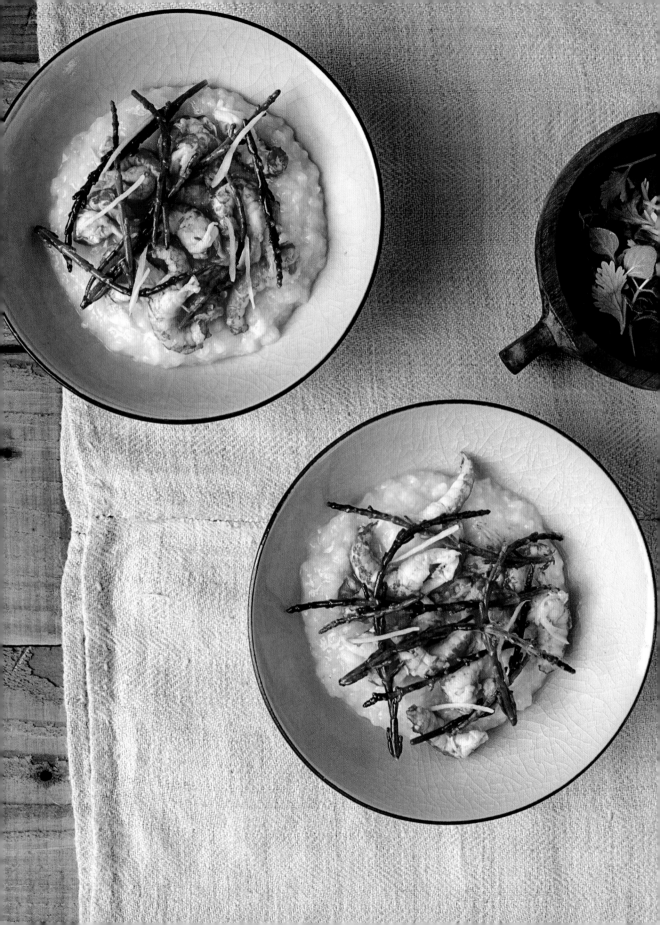

CRAYFISH CONGEE

SERVES 2

80g ordinary or basmati
  white rice
1 chicken stock cube
1/2 tsp ginger paste, or a thumb-
  sized piece of fresh root
  ginger, peeled and crushed
1 lemongrass stalk, bashed
unsalted butter, for cooking
100g samphire
200g cooked crayfish
fresh root ginger, peeled and
  cut into thin matchsticks,
  to serve
lemon juice, to serve

Congee is a Chinese way of cooking white rice in which the starch breaks down and you are left with a wonderfully satisfying base to which you add your ingredients, in this case crayfish and samphire. When you first make congee, its appearance does look odd, but it's similar to risotto and equally good. Congee works as a base for many ingredients, such as prawns, chicken or pork, and including some fresh ginger is always a good idea.

Put the rice with 7 times its volume of water in a large saucepan with the stock cube, ginger paste and lemongrass. Bring to the boil, then reduce the heat to a low simmer and cook for about 1 hour, stirring every now and then, until the rice has broken down and the texture is gloopy. It may look a little odd, but trust us!

Heat a little butter in a wide pan, add the samphire and cook for 2 minutes. Remove and set aside, then add the crayfish to the pan briefly, just to warm through.

Divide the congee into bowls and scatter over the crayfish, samphire and fresh ginger. Give it a squeeze of lemon juice and it's ready to serve.

KITCHARI

SERVES 2

100g green mung beans
1 tsp ground turmeric
¼ tsp asafoetida (optional)
½ vegetable stock cube
20g unsalted butter
1 tsp panch phoran spice mix
(to make your own, mix 1 tsp
each of black mustard seeds,
cumin seeds, fennel seeds,
fenugreek, black onion
seeds and store in an airtight
container)
juice and grated zest of 1 lime
flaky sea salt and freshly
ground black pepper
Greek yoghurt, to serve
cooked brown rice, to serve
(optional)
fresh coriander leaves, to serve
(optional)

Kate swore she would never make anything with mung beans, having always thought they were created only to make dieters suffer. Then she discovered kitchari, which is an Ayurvedic soup designed to help balance the body. Perhaps because it's so balancing, it tastes good too. Never say never...

Rinse the mung beans in several changes of water, then leave them to soak overnight. Rinse the beans again and put them in a saucepan with 1 litre water. Bring to the boil and add the turmeric, asafoetida and stock cube. Reduce the heat to a simmer and cook gently for 45 minutes to 1 hour, until the beans are soft.

Melt half the butter in a frying pan and add the panch phoran spices and lime zest. Fry until the aromas are released, then add to the soup along with the lime juice. Taste and season with salt and pepper, then add the remaining butter, put the lid on and let the soup stand, off the heat, for 10 minutes. Warm through, if necessary, and serve with a spoonful of yoghurt and cooked brown rice, if you like, then scatter with coriander leaves if using.

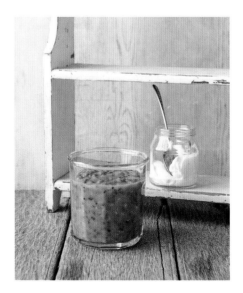

GARLIC SOUP

SERVES 4

3 tbsp light olive oil
4 garlic bulbs, separated into
  cloves but skins on
2 stems fresh thyme, leaves
  picked (you'll need about
  1 teaspoon)
1 tsp sweet smoked paprika
800ml hot chicken stock
  (page 14)
white wine vinegar, for
  poaching the eggs
4 eggs
4 slices ciabatta, toasted
flaky sea salt

Garlic has been a traditional remedy for thousands of years, and today we know that it has many beneficial properties, including being good for heart health and acting as an anti-inflammatory, antibacterial and antiviral. In other words, it's really good when you're feeling under the weather.

Heat the oil in a heavy-based pan over a low heat and add the garlic. Cook gently for about 15 minutes, or until golden brown. Remove the garlic cloves from the pan and allow to cool on kitchen paper. When cool enough to handle, squeeze out the soft centre of the cloves into a small bowl, discarding the skins. Return the pan to the heat, add the thyme and after a few seconds, return the garlic to the pan along with the paprika. Pour over the hot chicken stock, bring the boil, then reduce the heat to a simmer and cook for a few minutes to let the flavours infuse. Taste and season with salt.

To poach the eggs, bring a pan of water to the boil and add a splash of vinegar. Crack each egg into an individual small bowl or ramekin. Create a 'whirlpool' effect in the water by stirring it vigorously in one direction. As you do so, gently tip each egg from the ramekin into the middle of the water. Poach for 3 minutes, then remove with a slotted spoon and drain on kitchen paper. Divide the garlic soup between bowls and add a poached egg to each one, then serve with the toasted ciabatta.

EMMA'S CHINESE CHICKEN SOUP FOR FERTILITY

SERVES 4-6

1 small organic chicken
(weighing about 1kg)
4 cloves
1 tsp coriander seeds
5 cardamom pods, bashed
2 star anise pods
a few slices of fresh root ginger
3 strips *huang qi* (astragalus)
2 *dang gui* roots (angelica)
500ml black glutinous rice
wine, such as Shaoxing
noodles or cooked rice, to
serve (optional)
tenderleaf salad, to serve

This soup is unashamedly for women. Our friend Emma Cannon is an amazing acupuncturist and fertility specialist; she gave us this recipe, telling us: 'this is the Queen of soups. As one of my old teachers would say, even the making of it is something of a ritual; it's not only about eating but also connecting to the essence of the bones and heart of ourselves.' Gathering the ingredients, putting them in a big pot and watching the transformation take place is a bit like alchemy. It contains the Chinese herbs *dang gui* (angelica root) and *huang qi* (astralgus), both of which are gentle tonics that help to balance the female hormones. They are widely available in Asian stores or online (see Resources page 231).

Note: It is not recommended to include *dang gui* root if you are taking the medication Warfarin.

Bring a large pan of water to the boil. Add the chicken and blanch it for 5 minutes, then remove, drain and rinse it. Return it to the pot.

Put the spices, ginger and Chinese herbs in a square of muslin or cheesecloth and tie it up to make a spice bag. Add it to the pot along with the rice wine and enough water to cover the chicken. Simmer gently over a low heat for up to 4 hours, until tender.

Remove the chicken from the broth, allow to cool slightly, then take the meat off the bones, discarding the bones. Remove the spice bag and pass the stock through muslin or a fine-meshed sieve. Shred the chicken into large pieces by hand and return it to the broth. You can add your favourite noodles or ladle the soup over cooked rice, or just enjoy the simplicity of chicken soup on its own. Serve with the tenderleaf salad.

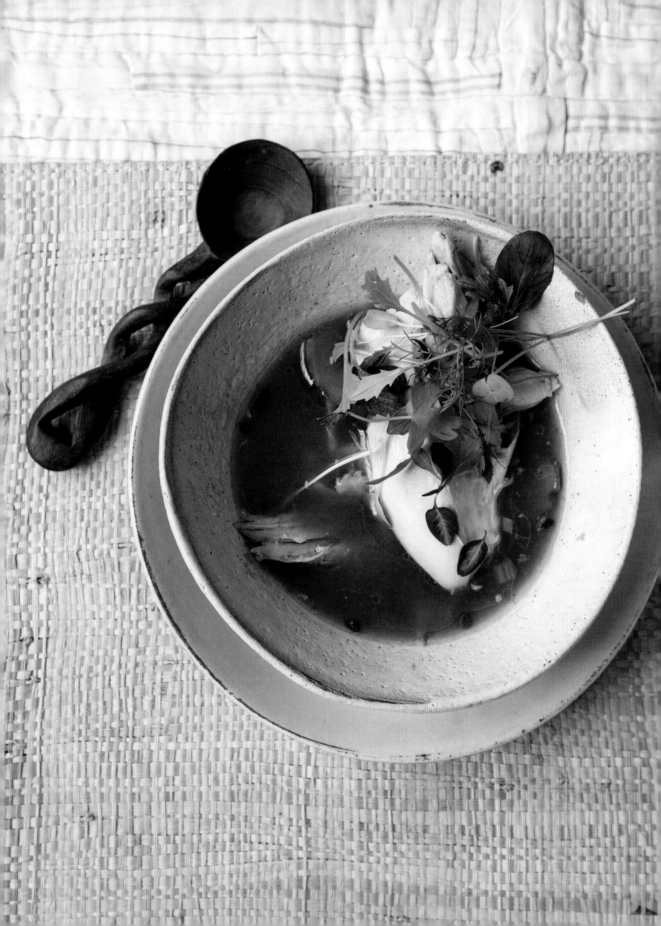

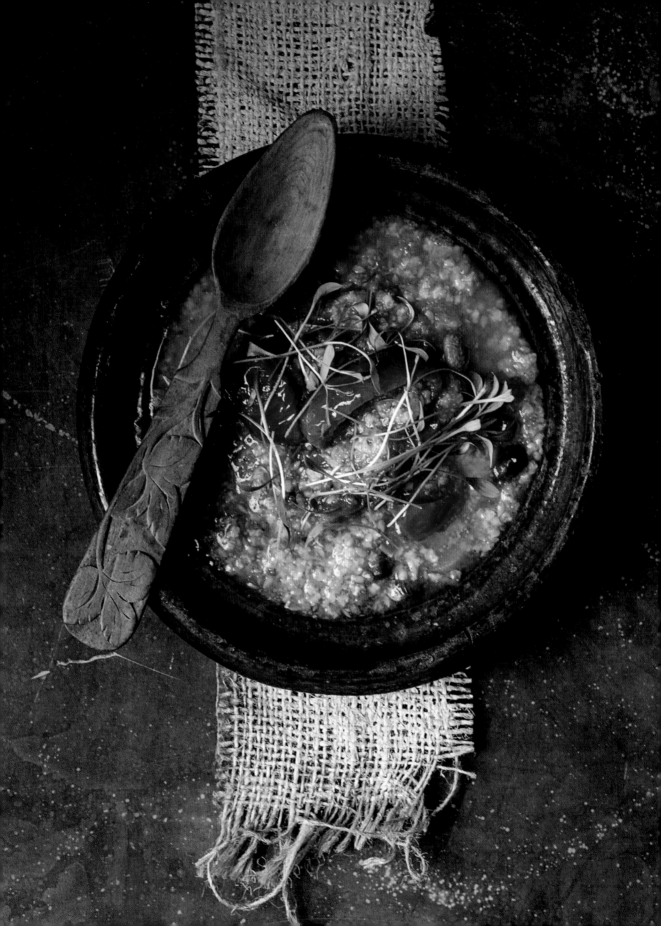

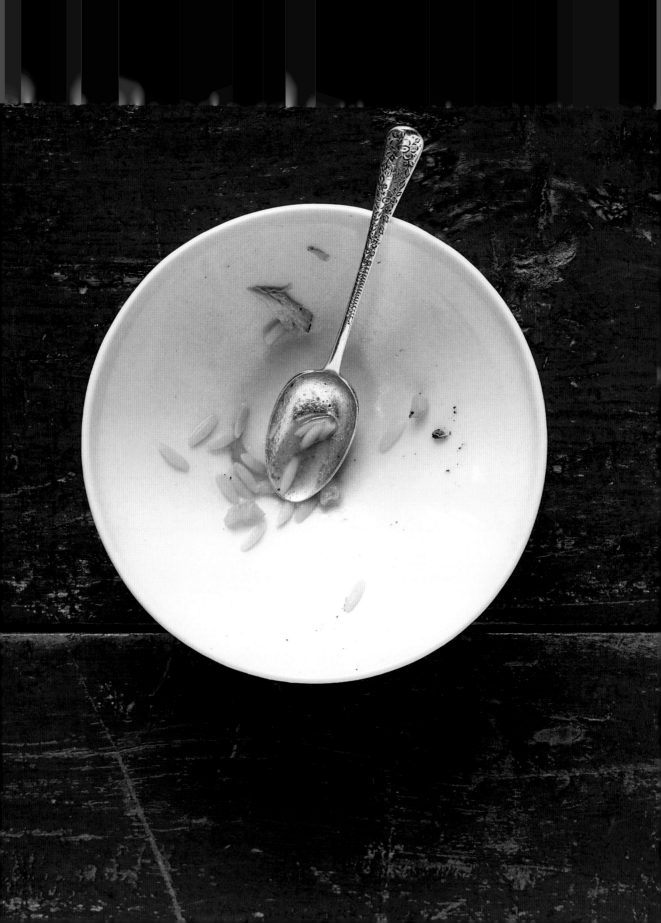

COCONUT PRAWN

SERVES 2

1 tsp white miso paste
200ml tinned coconut milk
1 lemongrass stalk, bashed
a 2cm piece fresh root ginger,
    peeled
4–6 kaffir lime leaves
1 green chilli, seeds removed
    and thinly sliced
grated zest and juice of 1/2 lime
1 tsp fish sauce
1 tsp mirin
100g udon noodles
10 raw North Atlantic prawns,
    with heads and shells
200g pak choi, shredded
1–2 spring onions, thinly sliced
handful beansprouts
tamari (soy) sauce, to serve

Despite the long ingredients list, this is basically a storecupboard soup that takes 10 minutes to make, and all in one pot too. The results are so fresh and vibrant, they'll brighten up any weekday evening. Furikake (see page 61) is a Japanese seasoning made with sesame seeds and seaweed flakes. It's a delicious alternative to sea salt, especially for East Asian dishes.

Mix the miso with a little hot water and then place in a saucepan with 200ml boiling water, along with the coconut milk. Bring to the boil, then reduce the heat to a simmer. Add the lemongrass, ginger, lime leaves, chilli, lime zest, fish sauce and mirin. After a few minutes, add the noodles. Taste to check seasoning.

Prepare your prawns by placing each one flat on a chopping board and running a sharp knife lengthways along the prawn to slice it in half.

When the noodles are cooked – about 5–6 minutes (check the instructions on the packet) – add the prawns and pak choi. When the prawns have turned pink, the soup is ready to serve. Ladle it into deep bowls and garnish with spring onions and beansprouts. Squeeze over the lime juice and add a little tamari to taste.

ANCIENT AMARANTH

SERVES 2

1 tbsp unsalted butter
1 onion, finely chopped
1 carrot, finely chopped
1 celery stalk, finely chopped
1 garlic clove, finely chopped
75g amaranth
75g millet
1 tbsp flaxseeds
1 tbsp chilli-infused oil (or
    1 tbsp olive oil plus
    8 chilli flakes)
1 tsp sweet paprika
500ml hot vegetable stock
    (page 15)
50g sunblushed tomatoes
1 heaped tbsp sundried tomato
    paste
60g pinto beans, rinsed
    and soaked in cold water
    overnight, then rinsed again
coriander cress or leaves,
    to garnish
avocado, sour cream and
    natural corn chips, to serve
    (optional)

This simple soup is made very satisfying by the grains, beans and warming chilli and paprika. Amaranth (see page 28) is a tiny seed grown in South America which dates back to the Aztecs. You can use it a bit like polenta, or make porridge in the morning by simmering it in hot milk. We have combined it with a larger grain, millet, here, along with a spoonful of flaxseeds for good measure. A super soup.

Melt the butter in a heavy-based pan, add the onion, carrot, celery and garlic and cook gently for about 15 minutes, or until the onion is very soft. Add the amaranth, millet and flaxseeds, then stir before adding the chilli oil and sweet paprika. Allow to infuse for a couple of minutes, stirring, before adding the stock, sunblushed tomatoes, tomato paste and pinto beans. Bring to the boil, then reduce the heat to a simmer and cook over a low heat for about 40 minutes, or until the beans and grains are cooked. Serve with with coriander, avocado, sour cream and natural corn chips, if you like.

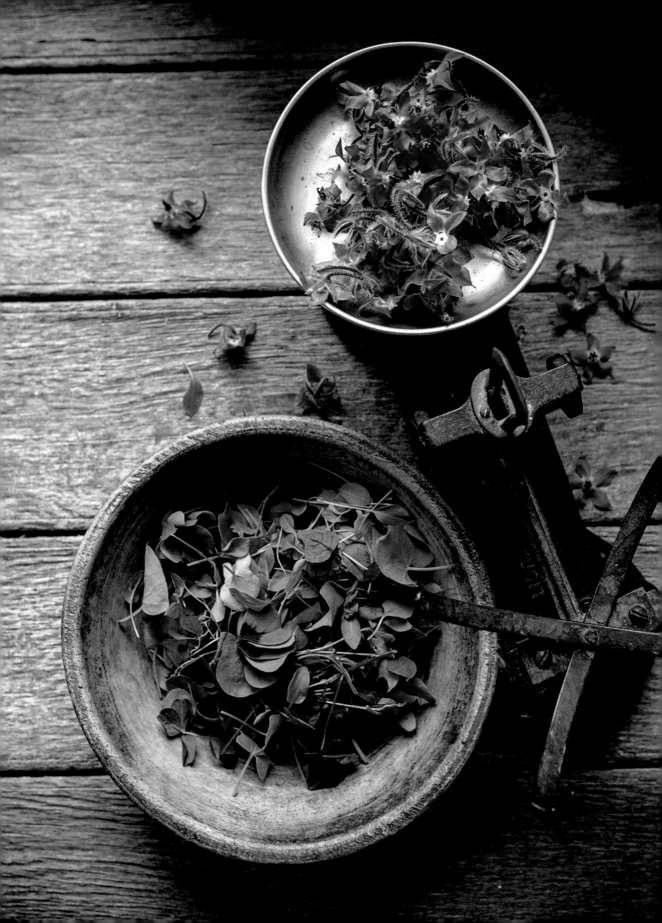

ROUND THE WORLD

'Memories are like mulligatawny soup in a
cheap restaurant. It is best not to stir them.'

P. G. WODEHOUSE, *WODEHOUSE ON WODEHOUSE* (1981)

Nothing recreates the memories associated with travelling to different countries and cultures better than food, which can bring back all the scents, sounds, sights and tastes of a place. Best of all, it seems that every country in the world has at least one unique soup that its inhabitants enjoy. We discovered the match made in heaven of Chicken, Lemon and Mint in Portugal and studied Vietnamese Beef Pho in the restaurants of Dalston in east London. The Greeks love their Avgolemono (egg and lemon soup) and the Swedish warm themselves with Sailors' Beef and Beer. At home, our desire for adventure can be nourished by trying out new recipes and flavours, discovering new ingredients and investigating how we can best use them. We don't always succeed, but that's the beauty of adventure: you never quite know what will happen from one day to the next but you can close your eyes and take the leap anyway.

AVGOLEMONO

SERVES 4

800ml chicken or vegetable
　stock (pages 14–15)
75g short-grain rice
2 egg yolks plus 4 eggs
juice of 1 lemon
2 chicory heads
15g unsalted butter
20g crisped rice, such as
　Rice Krispies
1 tbsp sweet paprika
olive oil, for frying
flaky sea salt

This is a southern European version of congee, the Chinese rice soup (page 109). The egg and lemon combination dates back to the Byzantine Empire and is still popular in Greek and Turkish cookery today. We could eat this all day, it's so good. The paprika crisped rice in this recipe gives just the perfect little bit of crunch on top. Try it!

Bring the stock to the boil in a large saucepan. Add the rice, reduce the heat to a very gentle simmer and cook, uncovered, for 20 minutes. Whisk the egg yolks and lemon juice in a small bowl and add a ladleful of stock into the mixture, whisking gently as you do so. Now pour this mixture into the saucepan with the rice, whisking gently and continuously as you pour. It will gradually thicken the soup slightly. Don't let the soup boil, or it will curdle. Shred one of the chicory heads and add, stirring well and continuing to cook for another 2–3 minutes. Taste and season with salt.

Meanwhile, melt the butter in a separate frying pan and, as soon as it starts to sizzle, add the crisped rice and paprika. Stir well to throughly coat the rice; when it is nicely coloured, remove from the heat and set aside. In the same pan, heat a dash of oil and fry the eggs for 2–3 minutes until cooked. Divide the soup among serving bowls, top with the remaining chicory leaves and the egg, then scatter generously with the paprika crisped rice.

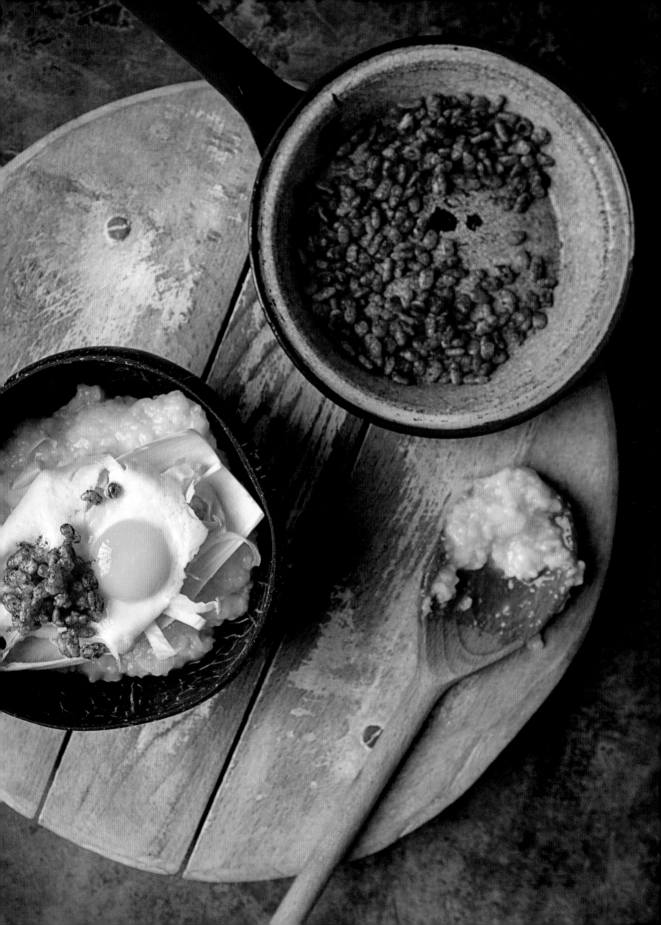

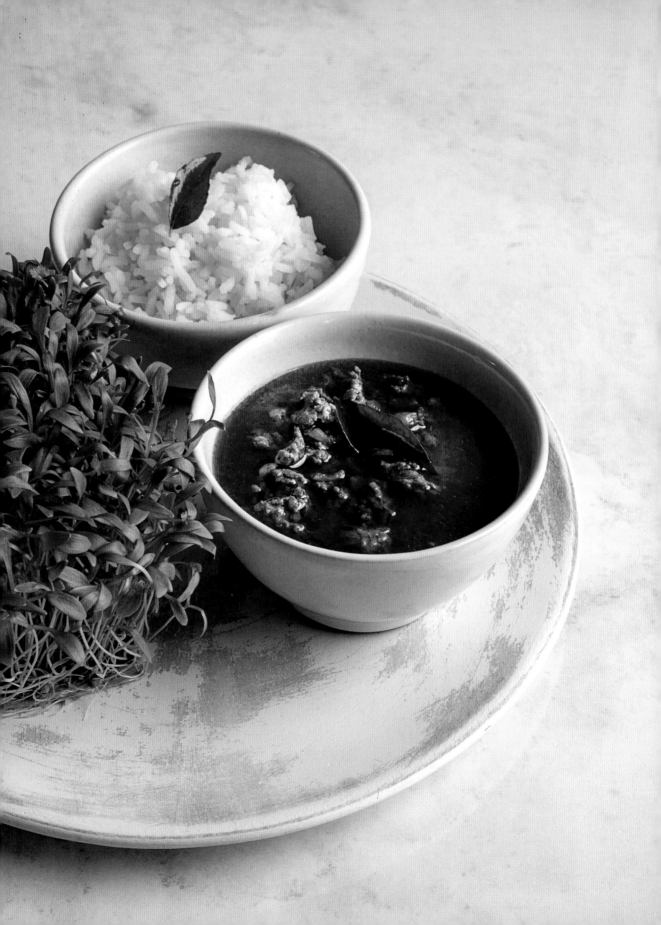

MULLIGATAWNY

SERVES 4

2 tbsp groundnut oil
1 large or 2 small onions,
    finely chopped
250g lamb or beef mince
1 tbsp garam masala
1 tsp ground turmeric
½ tsp ground ginger
1 tsp cumin seeds, bashed
    in a pestle and mortar
1 cinnamon stick
4 fresh curry leaves
1 bay leaf
1 green chilli, de-seeded and
    finely sliced (optional)
1 tbsp tomato purée
800ml beef stock (page 16)
100g cooked basmati rice
coriander cress or leaves,
    to serve
flaky sea salt

Mulligatawny is usually made with meat these days, as in our recipe here. However, in its original, simpler form it was true to its name, which is derived from two Tamil words: *molegoo* (pepper) and *tunnee* (water).

Heat the oil in a large heavy-based pan, add the onion and cook gently for about 10 minutes, or until soft, then remove and set aside. In the same pan, add the mince and cook, stirring occasionally, until brown. Make a space in the bottom of the pan and add the garam masala, turmeric, ginger and cumin seeds. Allow the aromas to release, then stir them into the mince, returning the onions to the pan at the same time. Add the cinnamon, curry leaves, bay leaf, chilli (if using), tomato purée and stock, give everything a good stir while you bring it up to the boil, then reduce the heat to a simmer and cook gently for about 1 hour. Taste for seasoning. Remove from the heat and allow to rest for 5–10 minutes. Serve the soup in bowls with the rice and coriander cress or leaves.

LIME & LENTIL SOUP WITH MARINATED FETA

SERVES 4

1 tsp coconut oil
1 onion, finely chopped
1 celery stalk, finely chopped
1 carrot, finely chopped
1 heaped tsp garam masala
6 curry leaves
200g green lentils, rinsed
750–900ml chicken or
    vegetable stock (pages
    14–15), depending on how
    thick you like your soup
1 tbsp tomato purée
juice of 1 lime
1 heaped tsp sumac
flaky sea salt and freshly
    ground black pepper

For the marinated feta

5 curry leaves
1/2 tsp each black mustard
    seeds, caraway seeds and
    fennel seeds
extra-virgin olive oil, for frying
100g feta, cubed

This soup will warm you on a chilly day. The marinated feta also makes a wonderful salad with heritage tomatoes in the summer. Although it is a fat, coconut oil is used by the body for energy rather than being stored as fat. It can take the heat of cooking (unlike extra-virgin olive oil) and is a good staple to add to your cupboard.

To marinate the feta, gently fry the curry leaves and seeds in olive oil to release the aromas. Add these to the feta along with the olive oil and stir well. Marinate overnight in the refrigerator, if you can.

For the soup, heat the coconut oil in a large saucepan or stock pot and add the onion, celery and carrot. Cook gently for about 10 minutes. Push the vegetables to one side to make space at the bottom of the pan and add the garam masala and curry leaves. Sauté gently until the aroma is released, then stir them into the vegetables.

Add the lentils, stock and tomato purée, and give everything a good stir. Bring to the boil, cover and reduce the heat to a simmer for 25–30 minutes, until the lentils are soft. Stir in the lime juice and sumac. Taste and season with salt and pepper. Serve immediately in deep bowls, crumbling and scattering the marinated feta on top.

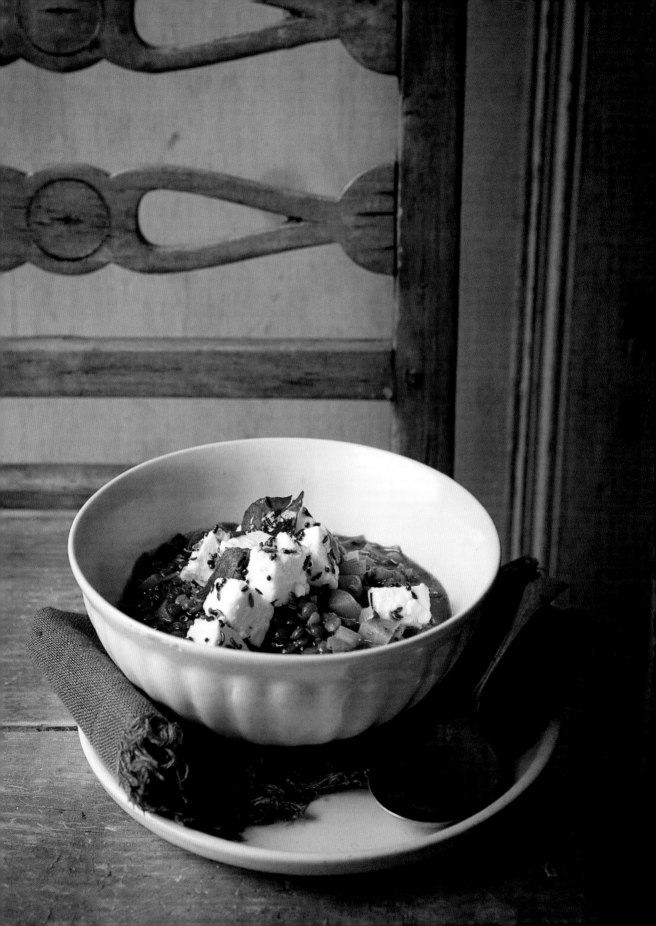

DAHL SOUP

SERVES 4

200g red lentils, rinsed
1/2 chicken stock cube
1 tsp ground turmeric
1 tsp garam masala
1/2 tsp mild chilli powder
1 tbsp unsalted butter
160ml tinned coconut milk
1 small onion, thinly sliced
1 tsp cumin seeds
1 tsp mustard seeds
1 tsp black onion seeds
juice of 1 lemon
flaky sea salt
full-fat natural yoghurt,
    to serve

This soup is perfect to fall back on during the week, as most of the ingredients will probably already be in the storecupboard. The essential thing to remember with spices is that you need to sauté them in a little oil before adding your other ingredients, as this releases all the aromas and flavours, and softens them so you don't get a harsh hit.

Put the lentils in a large saucepan with 3 times their volume of water and the stock cube. Stir in the turmeric, garam masala and chilli powder, plus half the butter and 1/2 teaspoon salt. Bring to the boil, then reduce the heat to a simmer. Add the coconut milk, cover and cook for about 20 minutes, or until the lentils are soft.

Heat the remaining butter in a pan. Add the onions, cumin seeds, mustard seeds and black onion seeds and cook for about 10 minutes, or until the onions are very soft and you can really smell the spices.

Add the lemon juice to the lentils, tasting as you go. Season with more salt if needed, too. Serve in bowls with the onions on top (or stirred through) and a little natural yoghurt.

HOT & SOUR AUBERGINE SOUP WITH WILD RICE

SERVES 4

2 large or 3 small aubergines,
    sliced into 3cm thick rounds
4 tbsp light olive oil
1 tsp flaky sea salt
1 cinnamon stick
3 cardamom pods
2 cloves
1 tsp anise seeds or fennel
    seeds
1 onion, chopped
1 fresh red chilli, de-seeded
    and finely sliced
3 fresh curry leaves
1 tbsp light brown sugar
1 tsp tamarind paste
1/2 tsp turmeric
100g wild rice, cooked
natural yoghurt, to serve

Aubergines have a reputation as being rather high maintenance, but this simple way of roasting them makes life easy and gives you soft, perfectly browned aubergines every time. Nicole has Yotam Ottolenghi and Sami Tamimi to thank for her love of them; Ottolenghi without aubergines would be like Italy without tomatoes.

Preheat the oven to 240°C/fan 220°C/475°F/gas mark 9.

Toss the aubergines in a large bowl with half the olive oil and the salt. Place in a baking tray and roast for 10-15 minutes, or until soft and starting to brown. Allow to cool, then roughly chop them.

Meanwhile, heat the vegetable oil in a pan, add the whole spices and cook until they release their aromas. Strain and reserve the oil. Put the spices in a square of muslin or cheesecloth and tie it up to make a spice bag. Heat the fragrant oil in the pan, add the onion and a generous pinch of salt, and cook gently until soft. Add the chilli and curry leaves and cook until aromatic. Add the sugar and continue cooking for 20 minutes until the onions have caramelised and you have a syrupy texture.

Return the spice bag to the pan and add the tamarind paste, turmeric and 500ml water. Bring the boil and reduce the heat to a simmer. Cook for 10 minutes, then add the aubergine and rice to the soup. Heat it through and serve the soup with yoghurt.

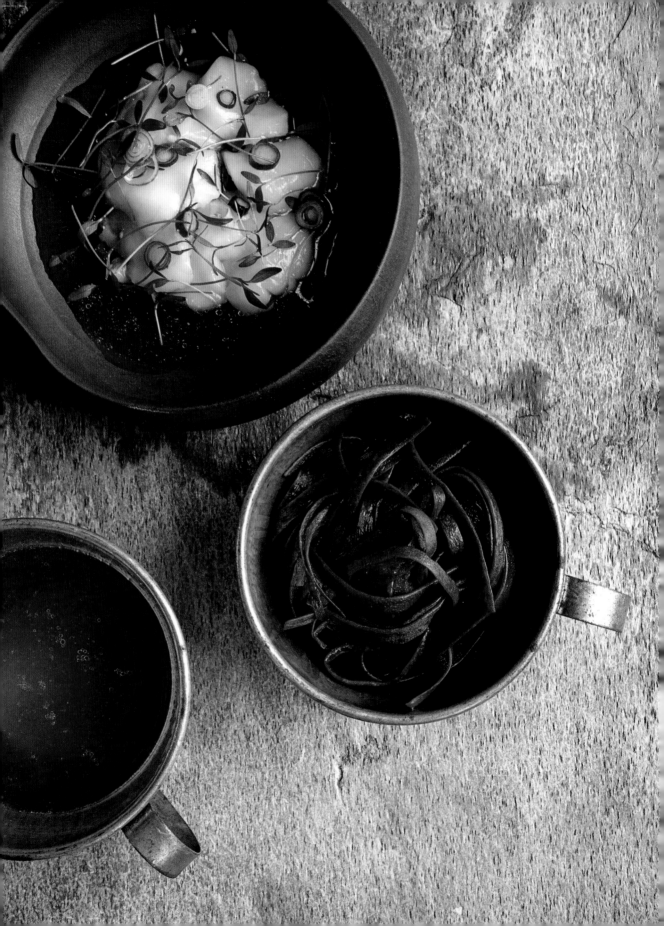

SEAWEED CONSOMMÉ WITH SCALLOP CEVICHE

SERVES 4

200g bacon, in one thick piece
    or lardons
1 tbsp maple syrup
3 small sheets of kombu
    seaweed
2 dried shiitake mushrooms
a thumb-sized piece of fresh
    root ginger, peeled
1 celery stalk, roughly chopped
1 carrot, roughly chopped
a handful of cherry tomatoes
5 egg whites, whisked
12 very fresh scallops
juice of 1/2 lime
20g sea spaghetti
a handful of fresh herbs such
    as red amaranth
1 spring onion, sliced
flaky sea salt and freshly
    ground black pepper

O God of the Sea,
Put weed in the drawing wave
To enrich the ground,
To shower us with food.

– Traditional religious Scottish chant

We tend to associate seaweed with Japanese cooking now, but it was once such an important part of the Scottish rural economy that ale would be poured into the sea to ensure a good harvest. Seaweed was used to help crops grow, to make soap and glass, and was eaten raw or cooked. It's packed with nutrients, in particular iodine, which helps thyroid health and promotes a healthy metabolism. So add a little seaweed to your life! Both kombu and sea spaghetti are widely available online (see Resources, page 231) and will last for years in your storecupboard.

Preheat the oven to 220°C/fan 200°C/425°F/gas mark 7.

If using bacon, cut into lardons. Toss the lardons in freshly ground black pepper and maple syrup, place on an oven tray and bake until caramel in colour. Add the kombu sheets to a large pan of water, along with the shiitake mushrooms, ginger, celery and carrot. Bring to the boil and add the bacon, cherry tomatoes and whisked egg whites. Simmer gently for 1 1/2 hours. The egg whites will form a solid crust on the top of the broth, which helps to clarify the stock. Remove from the heat and allow to rest before passing the liquid through a muslin-lined sieve. Discard the solids.

To prepare the scallops, slice them very thinly. Pat the slices dry with kitchen paper, then season with salt and a squeeze of lime juice. Cook the sea spaghetti according to the packet instructions until al dente.

To serve the soup, place slices of scallop in the centres of the each bowl, warm the consommé and ladle it over the top. Garnish with fresh herbs and spring onion and serve with the sea spaghetti on the side, for people to add to their soup as desired.

KIMCHI RAMEN

SERVES 1 (MAKES ENOUGH KIMCHI FOR 6)

For the kimchi
1 Chinese leaf cabbage
1 tbsp sea salt
25g Korean red pepper powder
50g Korean anchovy sauce
1 tbsp grated fresh ginger
1 tbsp garlic, thinly sliced
4 spring onions, finely sliced

For the ramen soup
70g ramen noodles
200ml miso stock
50g fresh silken tofu, cubed
1 spring onion, thinly sliced
1 tsp furikake seasoning
   (page 61), or sesame seeds

Fermented foods are enjoying a resurgence as people start to realise just how beneficial and friendly some bacteria are to our digestion. There are pickling traditions all over the world, from herring in Sweden to kimchi in Korea. We bought a kimchi kit online (see Resources, page 231), which has all the ingredients you need to make wonderful red, peppery jars of cabbage, plus a handy storage jar.

For the kimchi, shred the cabbage and separate it out. Toss the shredded cabbage with the salt, making sure it is evenly covered, and leave it to sit at room temperature for 4 hours.

Rinse the cabbage and drain it well. Mix the Korean red pepper powder, anchovy sauce and 50ml water to make a runny paste. Add the ginger, garlic and spring onions and pour the mixture over the cabbage. Mix it with your hands to make sure every shred of cabbage is evenly coated. Put the kimchi into sterilised glass jars, leaving some space at the top. Press the cabbage down so that enough liquid rises to the top to cover the cabbage. You may need to add a little water to the top. Seal the jars, making sure they are airtight so that fermentation can occur. Leave at room temperature for 1 day, at which point the kimchi will be ready to eat, or transfer to the fridge to store for up to a month.

To make the soup, bring a pan of water to the boil and cook the ramen noodles according to the instructions on the packet. Once cooked, rinse them in cold water, drain well and set aside. Heat the miso stock. In individual bowls, arrange 2 tablespoons chopped kimchi, the noodles and tofu before pouring over the very hot stock. Scatter over sliced spring onion and furikake seasoning.

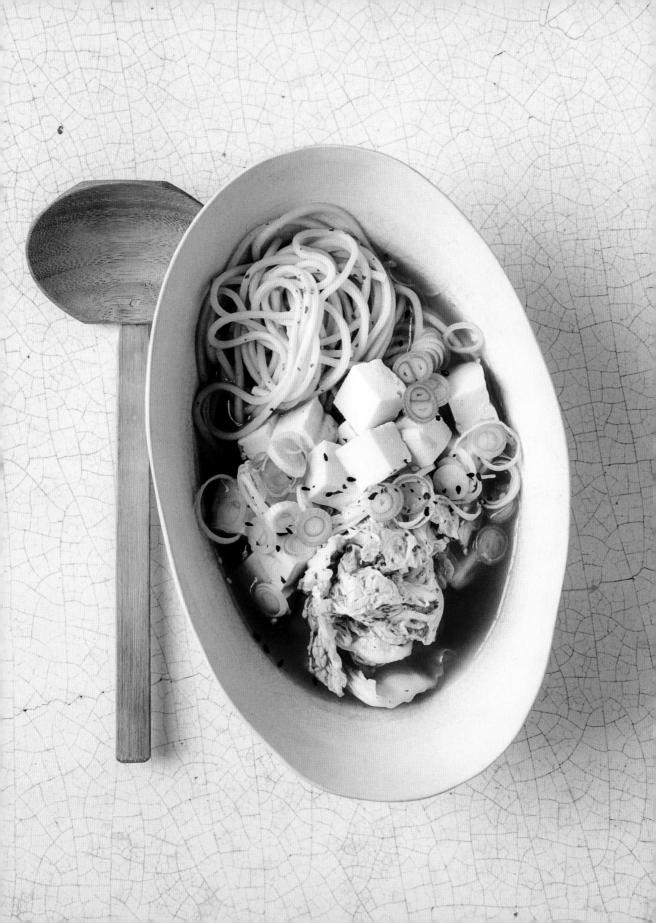

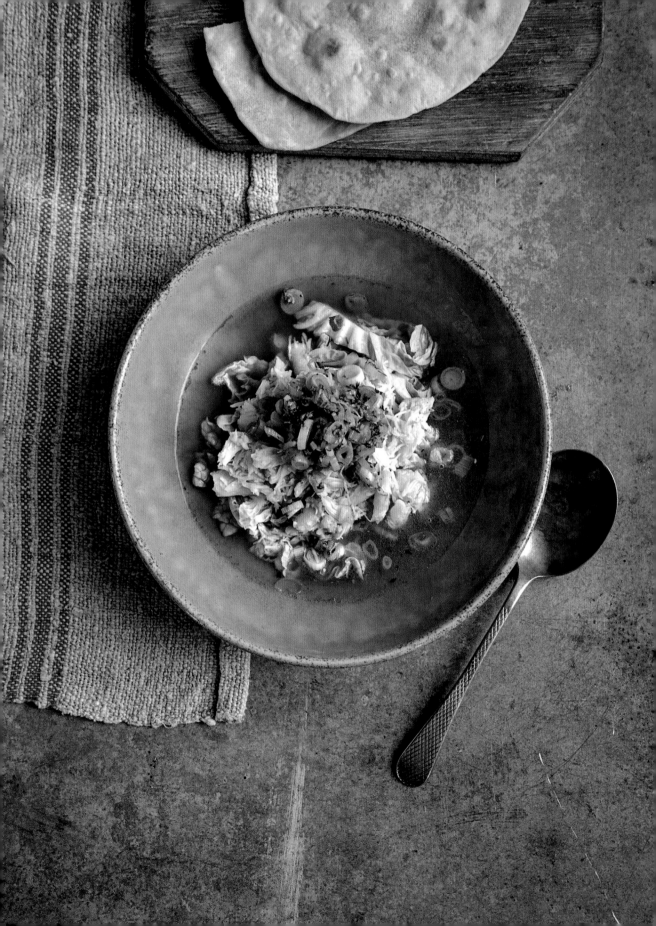

CREOLE CRAB

SERVES 2

1 tbsp olive oil
1 onion, finely chopped
1 celery stalk, finely chopped
500ml vegetable stock
    (page 15)
80g Chinese cabbage,
    shredded
100g white crabmeat
zest of 1 lime, grated, plus juice
2 spring onions, finely sliced

For the Creole spice mix
1 tbsp pink peppercorns
1 tbsp dried thyme
3 dried lime leaves
1/2 tsp garlic powder
1/2 tsp ground ginger

There are Creole cultures all over the world, and each one has its own language or patois, music, arts and, of course, cuisine. This Creole spice mixture is from the Réunion Islands in the Southern Indian Ocean, and contains pink peppercorns, thyme, kaffir lime leaves, garlic and ginger (see Resources, page 231). We thought why not add crab? The lovely aroma of this soup is like an ocean breeze. The recipe will give you more spice mix than you need but keep it in an airtight jar and use it as a rub for chicken or fish.

Make the Creole spice mix. Put all of the ingredients for the mix into a pestle and mortar (or use a spice grinder) and grind until you have a fine powder.

Heat the olive oil in a saucepan, add the onion and celery and cook gently for about 10–15 minutes, until soft. For the last couple of minutes, stir in 1 teaspoon of the Creole spice mixture.

Add the stock, bring to the boil and remove from the heat. Add the shredded cabbage and let it wilt for a couple of minutes. To serve, mix the crabmeat with another teaspoon of spice mixture and the lime zest and juice. Divide the crab among the serving bowls, making a high pile of meat in the middle. Ladle the broth around the crab and scatter over the spring onions.

ITALIAN WEDDING SOUP

SERVES 4

For the meatballs
½ white onion, finely chopped
400g turkey or chicken mince
40g dried breadcrumbs or
    panko crumbs
1 egg, lightly beaten
1 tbsp grated Parmesan cheese
2 tbsp light olive oil
flaky sea salt and freshly
    ground black pepper

For the soup
800ml chicken stock (page 14)
40g oregano leaves, plus extra
    to garnish
1 head radicchio, shredded
2 eggs
grated Parmesan cheese,
    to serve

You may not find soup being served at too many Italian weddings these days, but we like the idea of it! We think of soups as meals that bring friends and families together, sharing food and stories across the table.

To make the meatballs, combine all the ingredients in a large mixing bowl and season with salt and pepper. Roll into small balls approximately 2.5cm in diameter. Heat the olive oil in a large frying pan, add the meatballs in batches and fry until brown on all sides, then remove and set aside.

In a large pan, bring the chicken stock to the boil. Add the meatballs and simmer for 20 minutes, or until cooked through, before adding the oregano and radicchio. Whisk the eggs in a bowl. Stir the soup in a circular motion and while stirring, pour the eggs into the soup in a thin stream. Use a fork to gently create ribbons with the egg. Serve immediately with extra oregano leaves and grated Parmesan cheese.

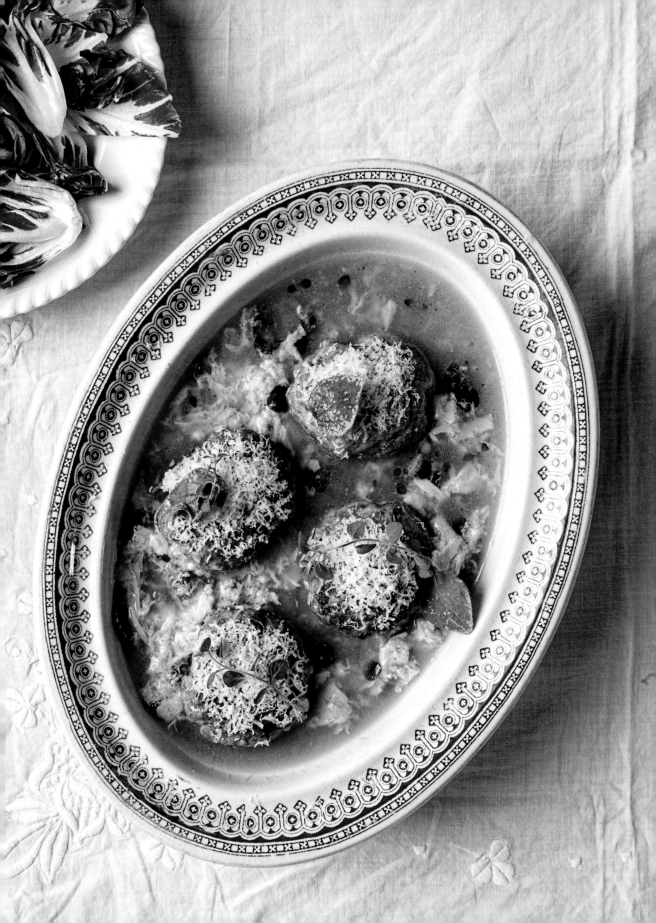

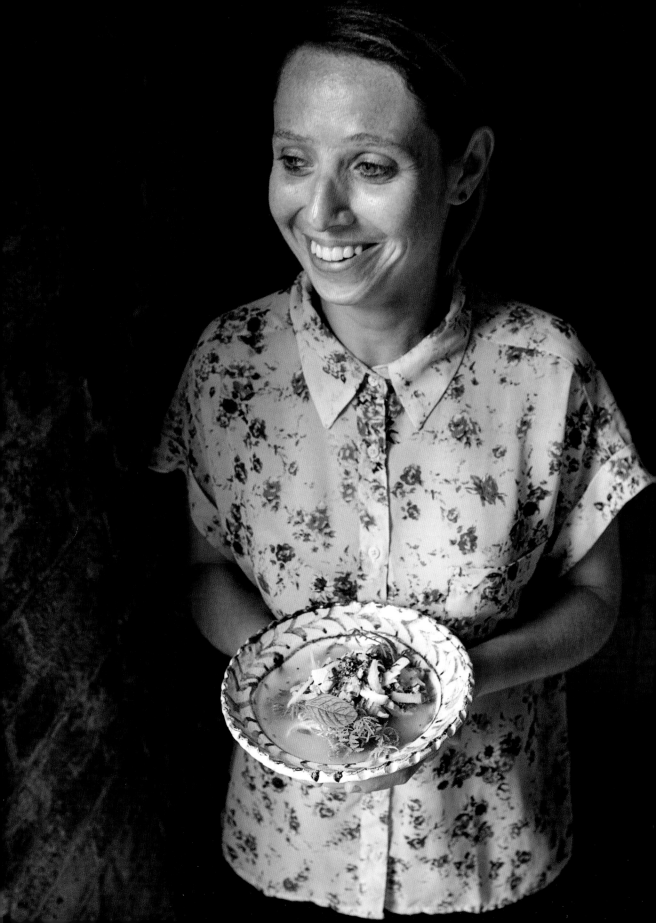

PORTUGUESE CHICKEN, LEMON & MINT

SERVES 4

2 litres chicken stock (page 14)

4 boneless, skinless chicken thighs

zest of 1 unwaxed lemon, cut into very thin strips

a good handful of fresh mint leaves, chopped

100g quinoa, rinsed

juice of 1 lemon, plus extra if needed

flaky sea salt and freshly ground black pepper

We first came across this soup in a little bakery in Tavira, Portugal, and fell in love with the comforting combination of chicken, lemon and mint. It's so simple to make, and always a winner. We guarantee you won't be disappointed.

Bring the chicken stock to the boil in a large pan, then add the chicken thighs, lemon zest and mint (reserve about 1 tablespoon for serving). Poach gently for 10–15 minutes, or until the chicken is cooked through. Remove the chicken from pan, leave it to cool a little, then slice or pull it into thin strips.

Bring the stock to the boil and add the quinoa. Simmer gently for about 15 minutes, or until the quinoa has puffed up and is tender, but still has a little bite. Return the chicken to the pan along with the juice of half a lemon. Taste to see if you need to add more. Cook for about 4 minutes then remove from the heat and add the reserved chopped mint. Taste and season with salt and pepper. Give everything a good stir before ladling into deep bowls, as the quinoa will settle to the bottom.

CHICK 'N' MASALA

SERVES 2

1 poussin
1/2 lemon, zest grated
1 tbsp tikka spice blend
1 tsp English mustard
1 tsp ginger paste (ready made,
  or crush your own fresh
  root ginger)
1/2 tsp garlic paste (ready
  made, or crush your
  own garlic)
1/2 tsp flaky sea salt
2 tbsp tomato purée
3–4 shallots, peeled and
  quartered
400ml hot chicken stock
  (page 14)
a bunch of fresh coriander or
  flat-leaf parsley
2 spring onions, thinly sliced

This is a lighter version of the classic curry, still with all the flavours. We use poussin because it gives you more surface area for the spice rub and is more moist and tender than chicken breast. We also favour a delicious ready-made tikka spice blend or to make your own, grind 1 tsp sweet paprika with 1/2 tsp each of fenugreek seeds, cumin seeds, hot paprika, coriander seeds, turmeric and garam masala, and 1/4 tsp each of cinnamon, chilli powder and caraway seeds, plus the seeds from 3 cardamom pods.

Preheat the oven to 180°C/fan 160°C/375°F/gas mark 4.

Pat the poussin dry with kitchen paper and rub it with the cut side of the lemon half. In a bowl, make a paste with the tikka spice blend, English mustard, ginger paste, garlic paste, lemon zest, salt and tomato purée. Rub the paste into the poussin and over the shallots.

Cut the wing tips off, then place the poussin on the shallots in an ovenproof dish. Squash it down a bit, then roast, uncovered, for 30 minutes. Transfer to the grill and grill it for 5 minutes until the skin has browned. Now pour the hot stock around the poussin. Cover it with foil and continue to cook in the oven for another 30 minutes. Turn the oven off and leave the poussin inside to rest, still covered with the foil. Serve in a large shallow bowl scattered with plenty of coriander leaves and spring onions, then pull the meat off the poussin and ladle over the broth and onions into individual bowls.

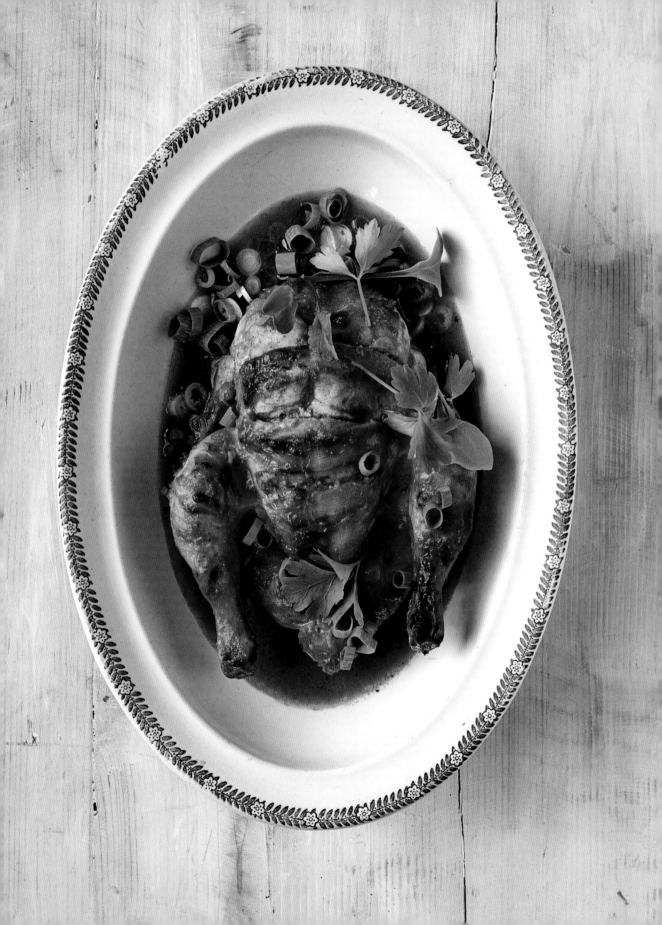

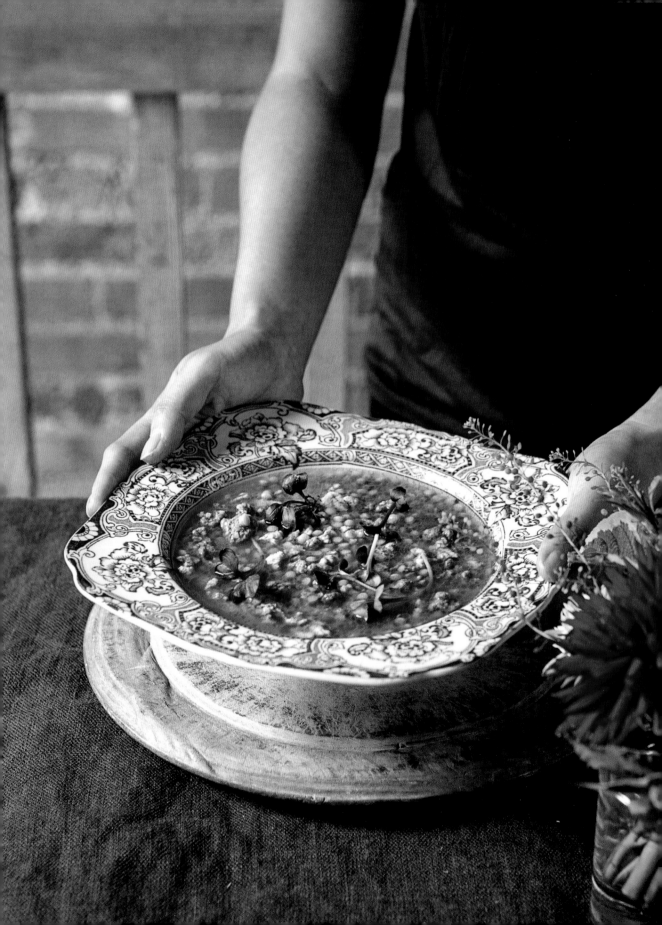

LARB GAI WITH GIANT COUSCOUS

SERVES 2

180g turkey or chicken mince
1 tsp Thai massaman curry
    paste, or other flavouring
    (see introduction)
500ml chicken stock (page 14)
80g giant couscous
a little groundnut or olive oil
8 curry leaves
1 tbsp chopped fresh coriander
red basil leaves, to garnish
    (optional)

This is such a versatile recipe: basically, mince, couscous and stock, to which you add the flavour of your choice while cooking the mince. You might fancy a Keralan curry paste, or ras el hanout or za'atar (see page 82) for a Middle Eastern flavour. Fresh herbs are always good too, especially basil or coriander. Giant couscous has a texture similar to pasta and is easier to use in soups than regular couscous, although either will work.

In a large bowl, mix the turkey mince with your choice of curry paste or spice and leave to marinate for 30 minutes. Bring the chicken stock to the boil in a pan and add the couscous. Reduce the heat to a fast simmer and cook according to the packet instructions – usually about 12 minutes.

Heat the oil in a large frying pan and and fry the curry leaves for 1 minute before adding the marinated mince. Fry until the mince is golden and cooked through. Add the coriander to the mince and stir it through. Drain the couscous, reserving the stock, and divide the couscous between the serving bowls. Top the couscous with the mince, then pour over as much stock as you like. Sprinkle with a few red basil leaves if you have them.

SWEDISH SAILORS' BEEF & BEER

SERVES 4

flour, for dusting
800g beef skirt or other
    stewing steak, cut into pieces
4 tbsp light olive oil
8 shallots, quartered
800g–1kg potatoes, cubed
500ml ale
4 bay leaves
200–300ml beef stock
    (page 16)
flaky sea salt and freshly
    ground black pepper

Leave this soup bubbling in the oven for a few hours while you take to the waves – or failing that, the countryside – to work up an appetite.

Preheat the oven to 150°C/fan 130°C/300°F/gas mark 2.

Season the flour with salt and dust the beef pieces in it, shaking off any excess. Heat the oil in a large ovenproof casserole dish, add the beef in batches and brown on all sides. Remove and set aside.

Add the shallots to the same pan and cook for 2 minutes, then add the potatoes. Give everything a good stir, then return the beef to the pan along with the ale and bay leaves. Add the beef stock and make sure everything is covered. Taste and season with salt and pepper if needed. Bring to the boil, then remove from the heat, put the lid on and transfer to the oven. Cook for about 4 hours, until the beef is very tender. Remove from the oven and allow to rest before serving.

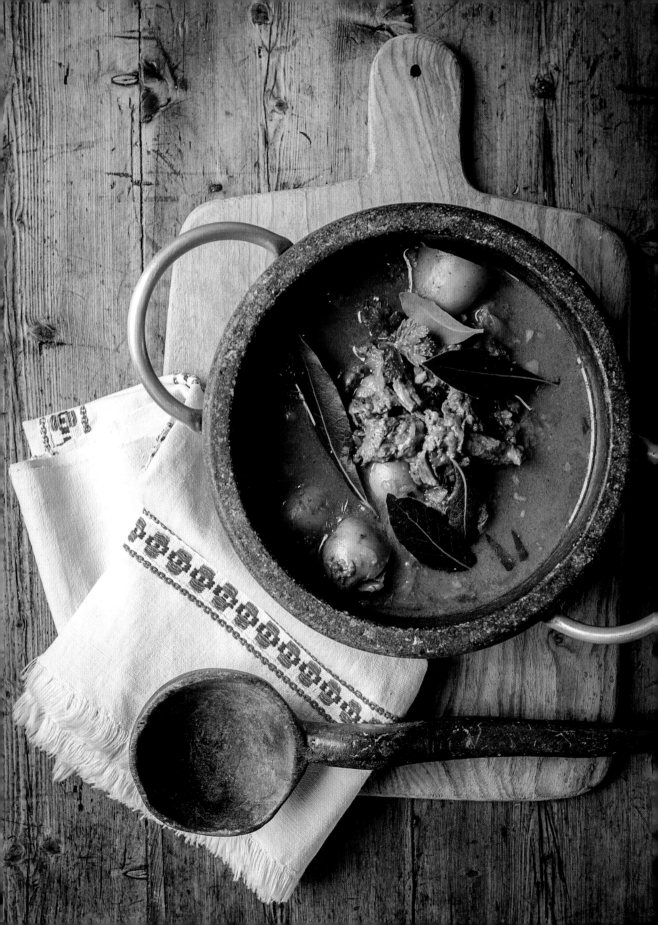

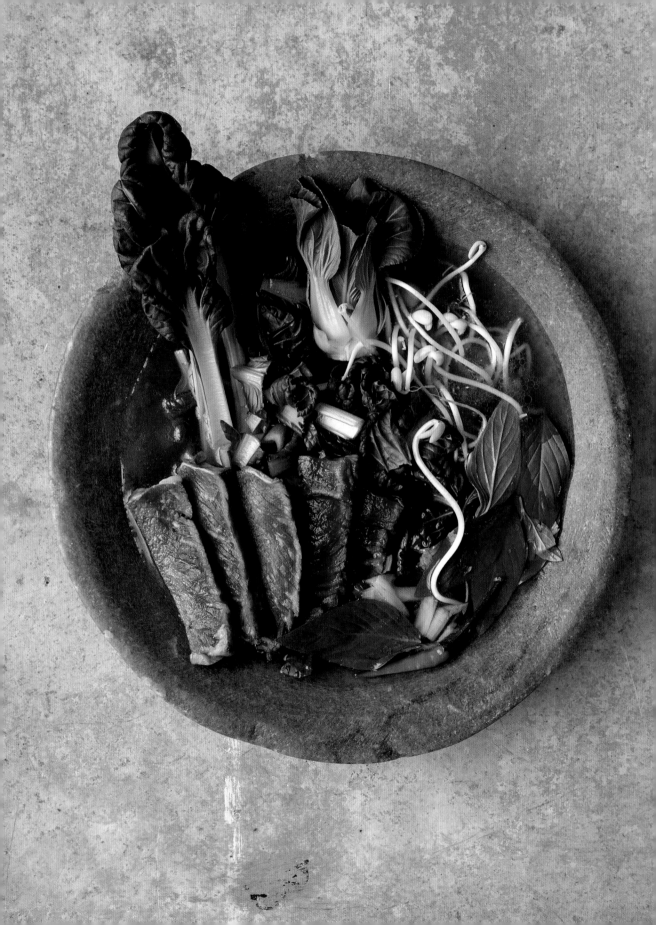

RIB-EYE PHO

SERVES 2

200g rib-eye steak
knob unsalted butter
400ml chicken stock (page 14)
1 star anise pod
1 cinnamon stick
1 lemongrass stalk, bashed
about 2cm fresh root ginger,
    thickly sliced
1 tsp fish sauce
100g baby pak choi, leaves
    separated
100g tat soi, or other Chinese
    greens, stalks chopped
1 red chilli
4 spring onions, thinly sliced
a handful of fresh lime basil
    leaves (or coriander)
a handful of beansprouts
flaky sea salt
lime wedges, to serve

Vietnamese is such a delicious cuisine, and very healthy too. This recipe is a bit of luxury, but we all deserve that! When cooking the steak, you need to be confident with the heat when you sear it, and then let it rest properly. That way, you can have melt-in-the-mouth rare beef with no blood. It's a treat, but a worthy one.

To prepare the steak, season it well with salt on both sides. Heat a ridged griddle pan until very hot and sear the steak for approximately 4 minutes on each side. The trick is to see when it begins to sweat; that's your cue to flip it over. Once the steak has seared, add a knob of butter to the pan and take it off the heat. Spoon the butter over the steak and allow it to rest while you prepare the rest of the pho.

Heat the chicken stock with the star anise, cinnamon, lemongrass and ginger. Bring to the boil, then reduce the heat to a simmer and cook gently for 20 minutes or so. Remove the whole spices from the stock and add the fish sauce. Add the pak choi and simmer for 2 minutes in the stock.

Slice the steak into thin strips. Divide among the serving bowls, then add the pak choi and tat soi. Ladle over the hot stock and scatter with the chilli, spring onions, lime basil leaves and beansprouts. Serve with lime wedges to squeeze over.

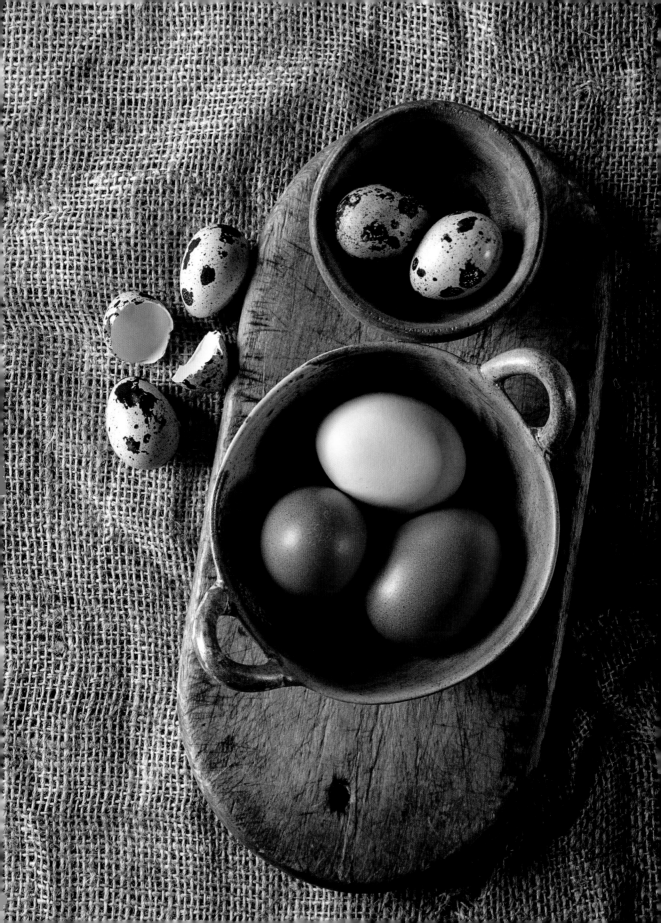

COMFORT

Made with love

Comfort food is made with love. It can be sunk into. It's soft at the edges, it fits your mood, and it can also makes things better. In her novel *The Particular Sadness of Lemon Cake*, Aimee Bender memorably describes a bowl of French onion soup that's nourishing in many ways: 'The smell took over the table, a warmingness … the taste of the soup washed through me. Warm, kind, focused, whole. It was easily, without question, the best soup I had ever had.'

For us, comfort is the cream of tomato soup Kate's mum gave her with Marmite sandwiches when she was little, or the Widow's Soup that Doris made for Nicole when she was growing up in Malta. We have also discovered new comforting soups to add to those from our childhoods; we had no idea peanut butter soup would be so good! We've added a few new twists and flavours to some old favourites in these recipes, and brought a little of our childhoods back with a few stars. We rekindled a love of corned beef hash, and Nicole added a touch of Malta to a classic minestrone. Grab a spoon and dig in: all these soups will make you feel good.

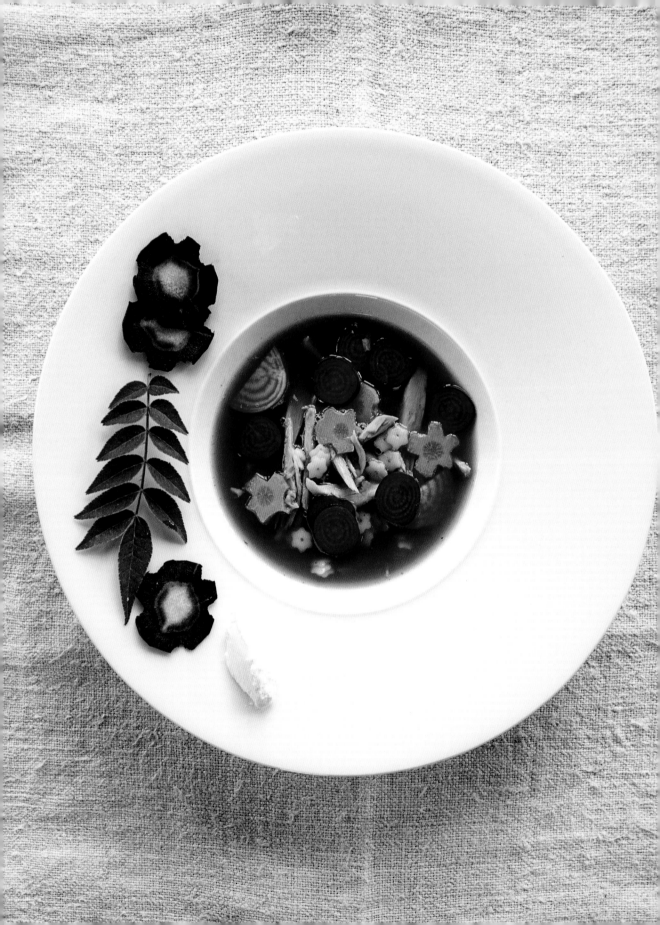

CHICKEN & STARS

SERVES 4

1 small organic chicken,
    approximately 1.2–1.4 kg
250ml Madeira
250ml port
6 kaffir lime leaves
1 lemongrass stalk, bashed
2 carrots, cut into thin star
    shapes (a canelle knife is
    useful for this)
4 beetroot (variations such as
    golden or candy globe are
    good), thinly sliced (optional)
200g stelline (star-shaped)
    pasta
flaky sea salt and freshly
    ground black pepper
crème fraîche, to serve
sichuan pepper leaves
    (optional)

There's a quote we love by Maya Angelou: 'Whenever something went wrong when I was young – if I had a pimple or if my hair broke – my mom would say, "Sister mine, I'm going to make you some soup."' This soup will make many things better.

Preheat the oven to 150°C/fan 130°C/300°F/gas mark 2.

Place the chicken in a roasting tin and roast for 2 hours, or until cooked through, and the juices run clear when the thickest part of the thigh is pricked. Switch the oven off, add the Madeira and port to the tin, cover with foil and leave it to rest in the oven for another hour.

Strain the liquid through a muslin-lined sieve and reserve it. Remove the chicken meat from the bones and shred it. Put the bones in a pan, cover with the reserved liquid from the roasting dish and add the lime leaves and lemongrass. Bring to the boil, then reduce the heat to a simmer and cook gently for 2 hours, before straining again through a muslin-lined sieve.

To serve, bring the stock to the boil, then add the carrots and beetroot, if using. After a couple of minutes, add the pasta and the shredded chicken. When the pasta is cooked (check the instructions on the packet), taste and season with salt and pepper, then serve with a dollop of crème fraîche and sichuan pepper leaves.

WIDOW'S SOUP

SERVES 4

1 tsp unsalted butter
1 onion, finely chopped
2 garlic cloves, crushed
1 potato, cubed
2 carrots, cubed
1 kohlrabi (use fennel if you
    can't find it), cubed
1 small cauliflower, broken into
    florets
2 celery stalks, sliced
1 tbsp tomato purée
1.2 litres hot chicken or
    vegetable stock (pages 14–15)
80g shelled broad beans,
    cooked
80g peas
a handful of fresh flat-leaf
    parsley, chopped
flaky sea salt
ricotta cheese, to serve
thyme leaves (optional)

Nicole always talks of Doris when she describes Widow's Soup, a traditional recipe from her home in Malta. Doris is a family friend who made Nicole happy with this soup. The name dates back to World Wars I and II, when men were away in battle and food was scarce. It was made with all the vegetables you could grow in your garden and topped with local cheese (goat's cheese from the tiny island of Gozo is some of the best in the world).

Melt the butter in a large saucepan, add the onion and garlic and cook gently until soft. Add the potato, carrots, kohlrabi, cauliflower and celery and sauté for 2 minutes. Combine the tomato purée with a little hot stock and add it to the vegetables. Add enough stock to cover the vegetables, bring to the boil, reduce the heat to a simmer and cook for 10–15 minutes, until vegetables are just cooked. Taste and season with salt if needed.

Add the beans and peas and allow to heat through for a couple of minutes before adding the parsley. To serve, place a spoonful of ricotta in each serving bowl, then ladle the hot soup over the top and garnish with some thyme leaves if you like.

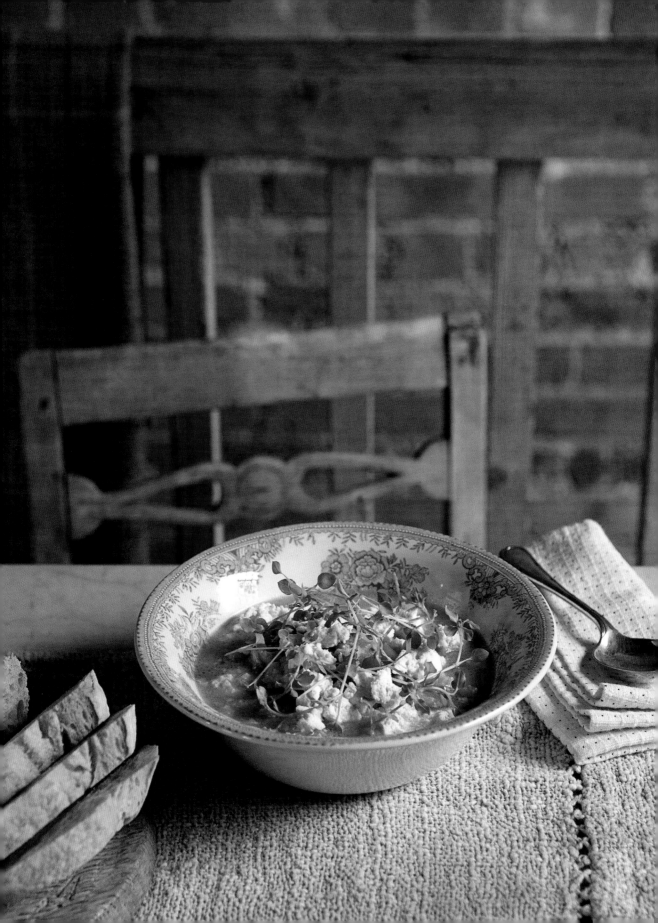

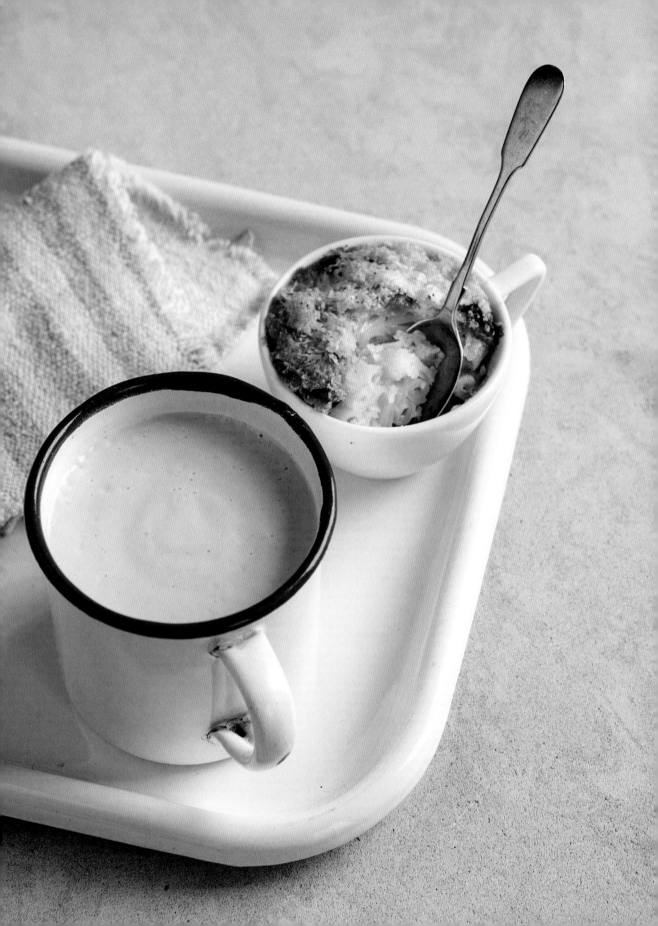

CAULIFLOWER SOUP & MACARONI CHEESE

SERVES 4

1 tsp sesame oil
500g cauliflower florets
500ml soya milk
½ chicken or vegetable
    stock cube

For the mini macaroni cheese
unsalted butter, for the
    ramekins
50g macaroni
25g strong Cheddar cheese
50g mascarpone
25g taleggio cheese
½ tsp hot wasabi paste
1 egg yolk
flaky sea salt and freshly
    ground black pepper

Most of the soups in this book are good for your waistline, but macaroni cheese is the yang to our yin, because for us, life without cheese wouldn't really count. We believe in mindful eating, rather than faddy eating, and in caring about what we put into our bodies. We do treat ourselves, regularly, and this seems to work out better in the long run than trying to restrict ourselves so much that we overindulge.

Preheat the oven to 190°C/fan 170°C/375°F/gas mark 5 and butter 4 ramekins. Bring a large saucepan of water to boil, add the macaroni and give it a good stir. Cook for 10-12 minutes (check the packet instructions), then drain well. Grate the Cheddar into a large bowl and add the mascarpone. Dice the taleggio into small cubes and add it to the bowl. Add the macaroni to the bowl while still hot; this will melt the cheese. Stir continuously. Add the wasabi and egg yolk and season with salt and pepper. Spoon the macaroni cheese into the ramekins and place in a bain marie (an ovenproof dish filled with enough hot water to come half way up the ramekins). Bake in the oven for about 20 minutes, until the tops are golden and bubbling.

Meanwhile, make the soup. Heat the sesame oil in a large saucepan or wok, add the cauliflower florets and cook for 1-2 minutes. Add the soya milk and stock cube and bring to the boil. Reduce the heat to a simmer and cook the cauliflower for 5-10 minutes, until you can pierce it easily with a sharp knife. Process with a blender until smooth, taste and season with salt and pepper. Serve with the macaroni cheese.

FRENCH ONION SOUP

SERVES 4

80g unsalted butter
800g small white onions,
    thinly sliced
2 tsp brown sugar
1 tbsp spelt or plain flour
100ml sake
1 litre beef stock (page 16)
3 large sprigs fresh thyme
2 bay leaves
flaky sea salt and freshly
    ground black pepper
wedges of sourdough bread,
    to serve

Traditionally, French onion soup is served with melted Gruyère croutons. For a change, we sieve the soup and serve it as a broth with a wedge of fresh sourdough bread and butter. We've also gone for a little sake to cut through the sweet onions.

Melt the butter in a large, heavy-based saucepan over a low heat and add the onions. Soften very slowly for about 1 1/2 hours, stirring occasionally, until golden in colour and beginning to caramelise. Add half the sugar to help the onions caramelise further for another 10 minutes or so. You can increase the heat a little at this stage.

Stir in the flour and half the sake, scraping any bits off the bottom of the pan. Stir in the rest of the sake and the beef stock. Tie the thyme and bay leaves together with string and add them to the pan. Bring to the boil, then reduce the heat to a simmer and cook for about 1 hour. Taste and season with salt and pepper.

Strain the onion broth and set aside the onions. Heat a small frying pan, add the onions and the remaining sugar and cook for 10–15 minutes until they form a chutney-like consistency. Warm the onion broth and serve with sourdough bread and the onions on the side.

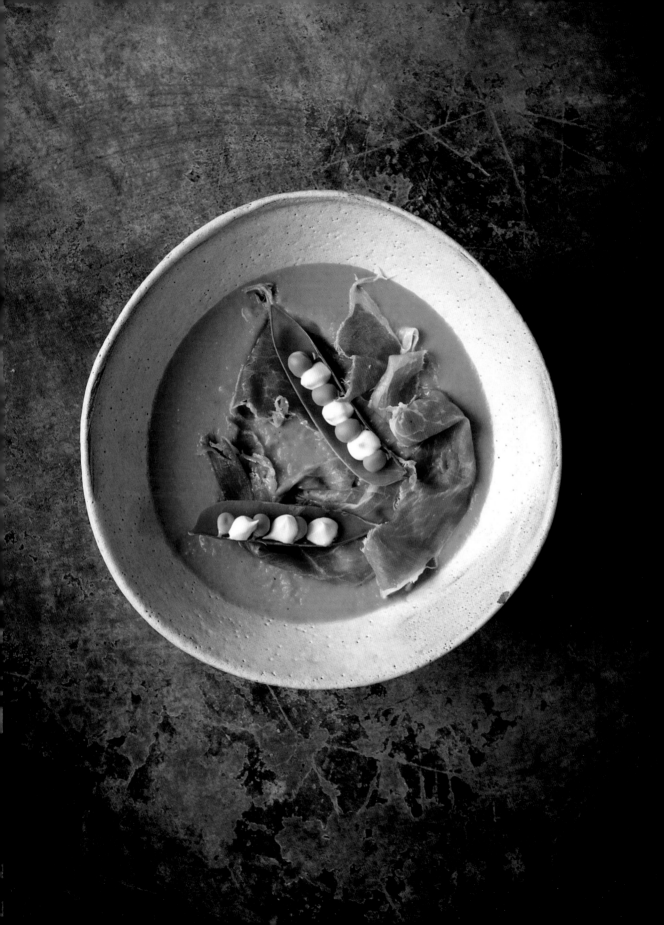

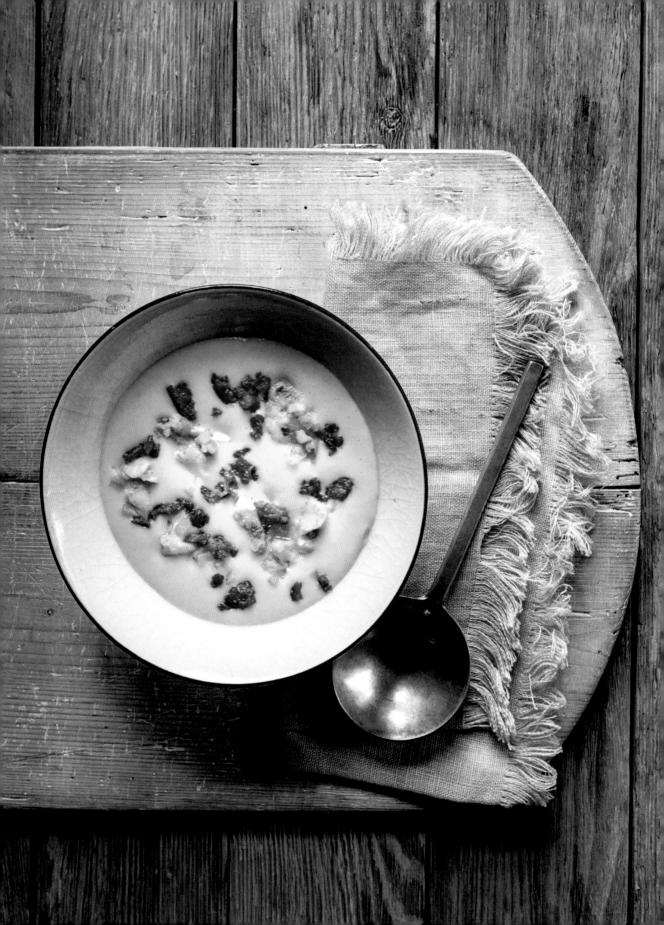

CORN, COD & CHORIZO

SERVES 2

200g cod fillet, in one piece
1 tsp ground turmeric
½ tsp flaky sea salt
½ onion, grated
40g unsalted butter
250g frozen sweetcorn
about 300ml whole milk
60g cooking chorizo, crumbled
   or sliced
1 tbsp light olive oil
flaky sea salt

Corn soup is very heart-warming; it's sweet, comforting and the kind of food that takes you back to your childhood. We've made it grown up with the addition of cod and chorizo. Sometimes the good things in life also come in threes.

In a bowl, combine the cod with the turmeric, salt and grated onion and leave to marinate in the refrigerator for 10 minutes (you'll discard the onion before cooking the cod, but it helps to deepen the flavour).

In a heavy-based pan, heat half the butter and add the sweetcorn. Cook gently until tender, adding a little water to make a spreadable consistency if the corn doesn't have enough residual liquid of its own. Process in batches in a blender, adding the milk until you have reached your desired consistency (we like this soup to be quite thick so that the cod and chorizo can almost sit on top). For a smoother soup, pass through a fine sieve before returning to the pan. Season with salt if needed.

Heat a small frying pan and add the crumbled chorizo; it has enough of its own fat so you don't need to add any more to the pan. Fry it until slightly crispy, then set aside.

Remove the cod from the marinade, scraping off the onion. In a larger frying pan, heat the oil until nice and hot, then pan-fry the cod for about 5 minutes. Add the remaining butter, turn the fillet over and remove from the heat. You should be able to flake the fish easily into bite-size pieces. Heat the corn soup through and ladle it into bowls, then divide the cod and chorizo between them and serve.

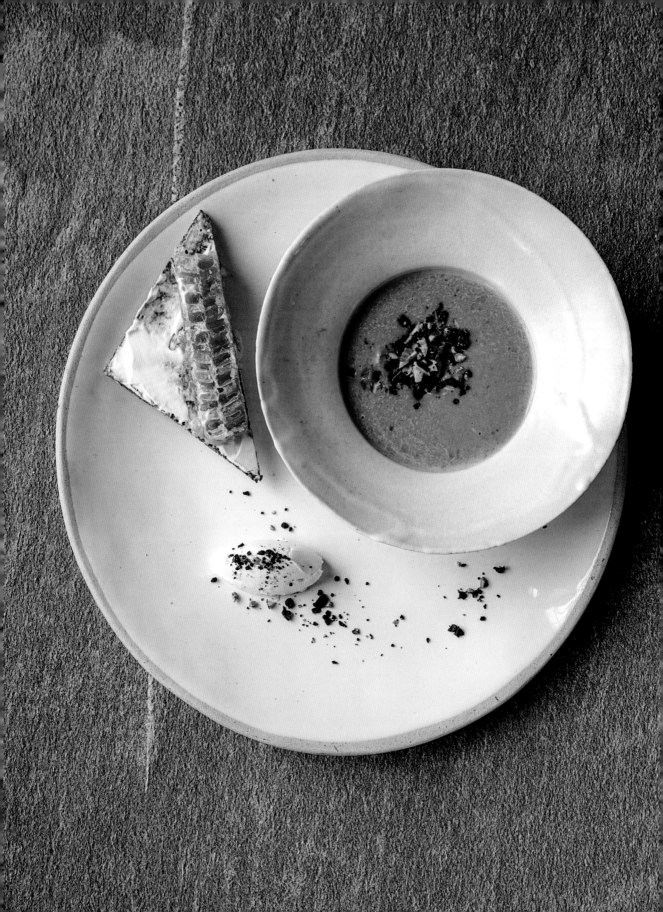

SQUASH & PEANUT BUTTER

SERVES 4

1 butternut squash
2 carrots (scrubbed if organic,
    peeled if not)
1 tbsp groundnut oil
1 litre hot vegetable or chicken
    stock (pages 14–15)
3 tbsp crunchy peanut butter
1 tsp bitter orange spice
    (optional)
2 tbsp charcoal peanuts or
    unsalted roasted peanuts,
    chopped
2 tbsp Greek yoghurt
flaky sea salt and freshly
    ground black pepper
honeycomb, to serve

If you like peanut butter, even if only a little bit, you'll love this soup. We've used a couple of special ingredients in this recipe and we urge you to try them: bitter orange spice has an interesting flavour – you can taste both the bitter and sweet flavours of orange side by side; charcoal peanuts are smoky in flavour and you can find them easily at Asian food stores. Ordinary roasted peanuts will also work well as a garnish for this soup.

Cut the squash into equal-sized cubes, removing the skin at the same time. Chop the carrots into similar-sized pieces. Heat the oil in a heavy-based pan and fry the squash and carrots until golden. Add the hot stock and peanut butter, bring to the boil, then reduce the heat to a simmer and cook gently for 20–25 minutes, or until tender.

Remove from the heat and stir through the bitter orange spice, if using. Allow to cool a little before processing in a blender to make a smooth soup. Serve scattered with the peanuts, Greek yoghurt and a little honeycomb.

MALTESE MINESTRONE

SERVES 2

100g spaghetti or short pasta
   such as ditalini
knob unsalted butter
½ onion, finely chopped
50g yellow beans
50g runner beans
50g green beans or snake
   beans
500ml vegetable stock
   (page 15)
50g fresh peas
Parmesan cheese, to serve
handful of pea shoots, to serve

For the green harissa
50g fresh flat-leaf parsley
1 tsp ground cumin
1 tsp ground coriander
10 cardamom pods, seeds
   removed
1 tsp salted capers, rinsed
   and drained
1 preserved lemon, chopped
1 garlic clove, crushed
150ml extra-virgin olive oil
a large pinch of flaky sea salt

Minestrone, a classic Italian soup, translates simply as 'the big one', and derives originally from the Latin verb *minestrare*, 'to serve'. There's no set recipe; it tends to be made from whatever vegetables are in season, often with the addition of pasta or rice. Nicole is from Malta, and this is her version of a minestrone. Malta stands on an underwater ridge connecting North Africa with Sicily, and its food is heavily influenced by its southern Mediterranean neighbour.

To make the green harissa, put all the ingredients in a food processor and process to a pesto-like consistency.

Bring a pan of water to the boil and cook the pasta according to the instructions on the packet, then drain well. Meanwhile, melt the butter in a pan, add the onion and cook for about 10 minutes, or until soft. In another saucepan, bring a large pan of salted water to the boil and cook all the beans for 3 minutes until tender, then drain well.

Heat the stock and whisk in 1 heaped teaspoon of the green harissa. Add the cooked pasta and peas and warm through. Ladle the soup into bowls and add the cooked beans. Finish with shavings of Parmesan cheese and sprinkle over some pea shoots.

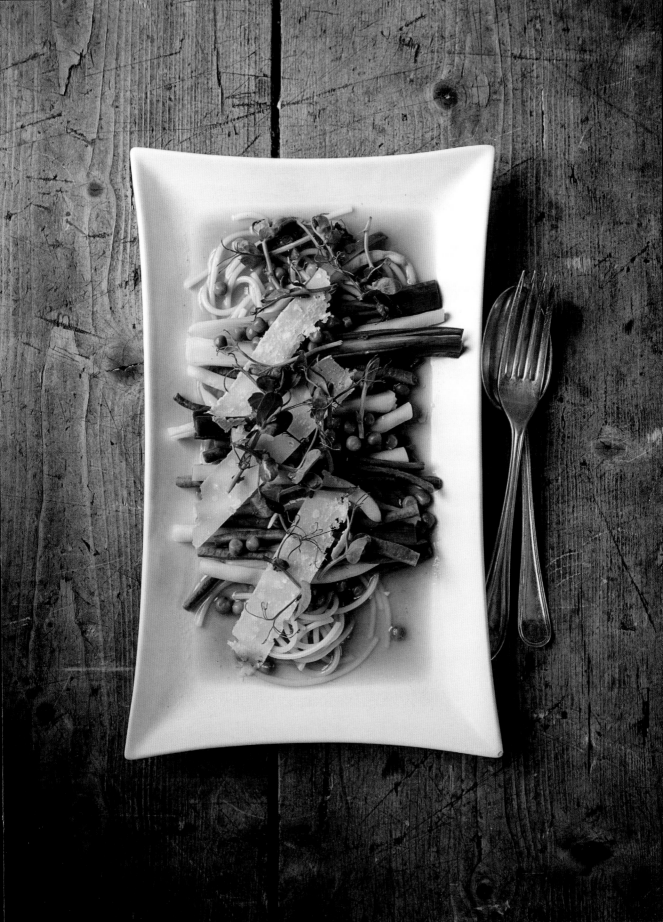

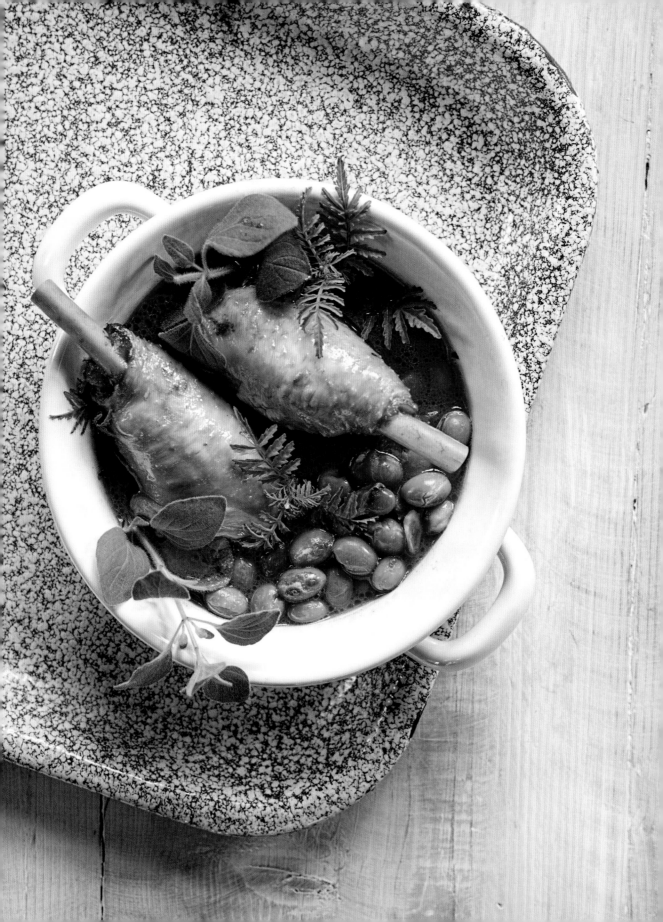

BIRD IN A BOWL

SERVES 2

groundnut oil, for frying
4 chicken drumsticks
500ml chicken stock (page 14)
1 garlic clove, crushed
1 bay leaf
1 tbsp tomato purée
400g tinned borlotti beans,
    drained
fresh sage leaves
flaky sea salt and freshly
    ground black pepper

Nicole mostly likes meat to be on the bone, and the same goes for fish. Why throw away all the flavour, the essence? Chicken drumsticks are great value and when you don't have the time or need to cook the whole bird, they are quick and easy. As kids, we both loved drumsticks because it was one time you got to eat with your hands, which really is the best way to eat them.

Heat a little groundnut oil in a pan, add the chicken drumsticks and brown them on all sides. Add chicken stock to just cover, along with the garlic clove and bay leaf, and poach the chicken gently for 30 minutes, or until the meat is tender and cooked through.

Add the tomato purée and borlotti beans, then season to taste with salt and pepper. Warm everything through before serving scattered with fresh sage leaves.

CORNED BEEF HASH, UMAMI
& A SMASHED EGG

SERVES 2 (MAKES 1 LARGE BOWL TO SHARE)

75g corned beef
1 tbsp finely chopped celery
1 tbsp finely chopped onion
1 tbsp finely chopped carrot
1 tbsp plus 1 tsp umami paste
    (available from large
    supermarkets or online)
1 tbsp tomato purée
1 tsp allspice
white wine vinegar, for
    poaching the egg
1 egg

Corned beef is from before time began (or at least from World War II), and umami is the newest taste to be discovered, which can be loosely translated from the Japanese as 'pleasant savoury taste'. If you are addicted to Marmite or Parmesan cheese, that's the umami. It occurs naturally in foods, and soups are generally thought to contains bags of umami, as the flavour develops in the pot.

To make the corned beef hash, crumble the corned beef into a large bowl and stir in the celery, onion, carrot and 1 teaspoon umami paste. Shape the mixture into a pattie and set aside.

For the soup, loosen 1 tablespoon umami paste in a little hot water. Add this to an additional 500ml hot water in a large saucepan. Whisk in the tomato purée and allspice. Bring to the boil, then reduce the heat to a simmer and cook for 10 minutes to allow the flavours to infuse. Pass through a strainer.

Bring a saucepan of water to the boil and add a small splash of white vinegar. Crack the egg into an individual ramekin or small bowl. Create a 'whirlpool' effect in the water by stirring it vigorously in one direction. Gently tip each egg from its ramekin into the middle of the water. Poach for 3 minutes, then remove with a slotted spoon and drain on kitchen paper.

To serve, place the corned beef hash pattie in the middle of a large bowl. Gently pour the umami soup around it so that the top of the pattie is still above the line of soup.

Carefully place the poached egg onto the pattie and use a fork to 'smash' it, just before serving. We suggest sharing one bowl between two people.

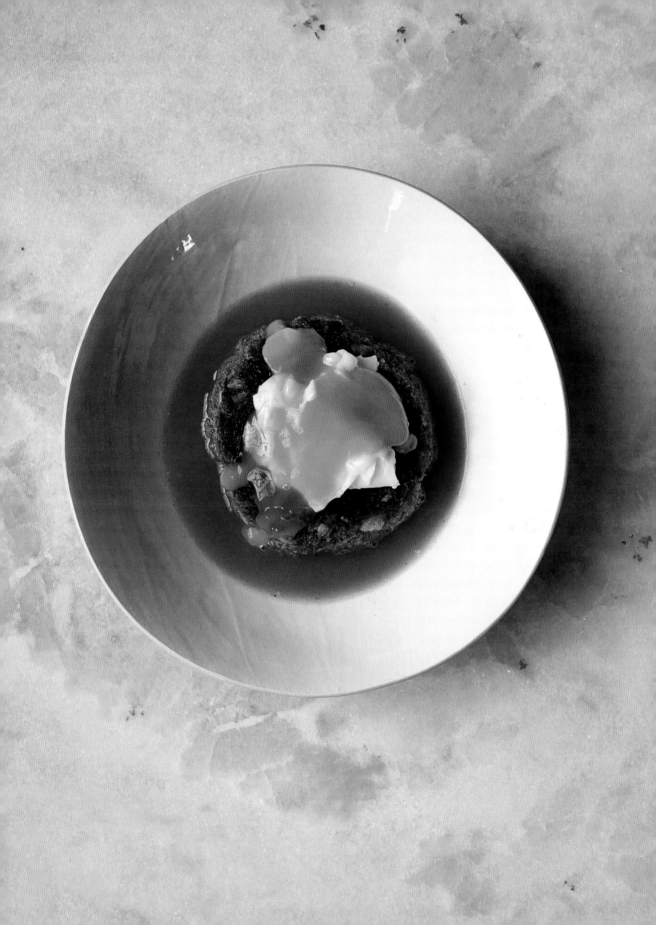

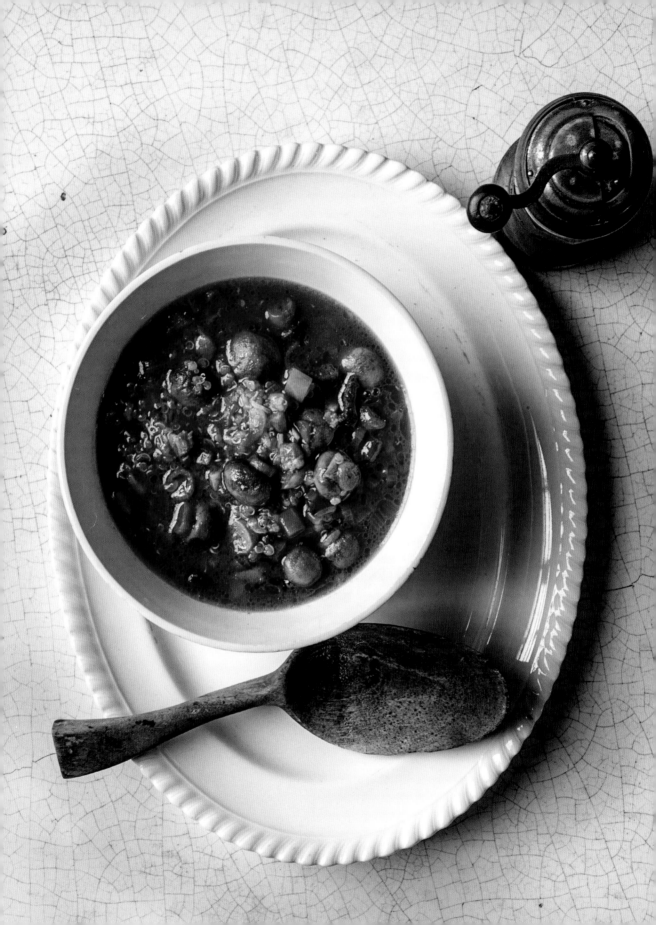

HOTCH POTCH

SERVES 4

1 tbsp sesame or olive oil

75g pancetta, chopped

1 small onion, finely chopped

1 celery stalk, chopped

2 carrots, chopped

2 garlic cloves, chopped

250g chestnut mushrooms, chopped

a small handful of dried porcini mushrooms (about 8g), soaked in hot water (or you can use any mixed dried mushrooms)

50g quinoa

1 tbsp tomato purée

a good splash of dry sherry

1 tbsp ponzu (or tamari (soy) sauce)

700ml hot chicken stock (page 14)

fresh flat-leaf parsley, chopped, to serve (optional)

The beauty of having storecupboard ingredients like tomato purée, quinoa, porcini mushrooms and tamari sauce is that you can make a delicious soup out of whatever fresh ingredients you happen to have to hand. We were never great fans of tinned mushroom soup, but this restores our faith not only in mushroom soup, but also in the blessed marriage of flavour between bacon and mushroom.

Heat the oil in a large, heavy-based saucepan or casserole dish, add the pancetta and sauté until browned. Remove the pancetta and set aside. Add the onion and cook gently for a few minutes before adding the celery, carrots and garlic, then continue to cook over a low heat for about 10 minutes until soft. Add the mushrooms, give everything a good stir and cook over a medium heat for 2-3 minutes, until the mushrooms soften.

Remove the porcini mushrooms from the soaking liquid, reserving the liquid, and finely chop them. Add to the pan, along with the quinoa, and stir well. Cook for 1-2 minutes, then add the pancetta and tomato purée and continue to cook for another minute before adding the sherry and ponzu. With the heat high, allow most of the liquid to evaporate before adding the reserved mushroom liquid and the stock. Cover and reduce the heat to a simmer for about 30 minutes, by which time the quinoa should be cooked but still a little al dente.

To serve, stir the soup well, as the pancetta and quinoa will have sunk to the bottom, then ladle it into deep bowls and scatter over the parsley, if using.

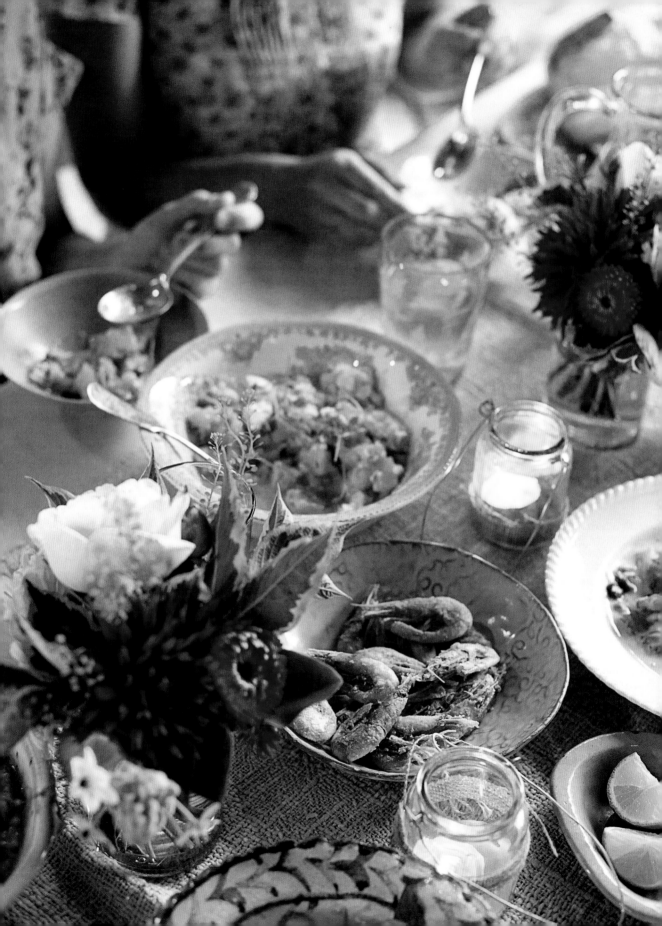

FEASTS

'Happiness quite unshared can scarcely
be called happiness; it has no taste.'

CHARLOTTE BRONTË (IN A LETTER, 1850)

These are soups that push the boat out. They require a little effort, but the time you spend in preparation nourishes and calms the mind after it has been in work mode. Some of them will take a bit of time and patience, but the depth of flavour you'll achieve is truly worth the wait. Our great passion is to see people sharing and enjoying food together, spending time in the kitchen creating something special and then putting everything in the centre of the table for friends to serve each other. Whether it's a Sunday lunch, dinner with friends or a family celebration, soups like the warming Braised Beef, Heritage Radishes, Baby Carrots and Horseradish Cream, or fragrant Thit Heo Kho will take the lead in the meal.

Our lifestyles might make it more difficult to gather round the kitchen table every day (perhaps that's why we increasingly seem to love going to food festivals), but food will always bring people together and give us something to get the conversation started. We hope these recipes and ideas will change the way people tend to think of soup, which is often as forgettable, or the option we choose because we're on a diet. Soups can be surprising, make us smile, eat too fast and feel happy.

AUTUMN BROTH

SERVES 4

4 portobello mushrooms
8 shiitake mushrooms
2 fresh thyme sprigs
1 bay leaf
2 garlic cloves, thinly sliced
500ml hot vegetable stock
   (page 15)
500ml white wine
6 tbsp balsamic vinegar
100g unsalted butter
200g mixed wild mushrooms,
   such as girolles, oyster,
   chestnut, enoki or shimejii
flaky sea salt and freshly
   ground black pepper

The easiest way to clean mushrooms is with a soft brush. If storing them, wrap them loosely in newspaper. Check out any farmers' markets close to you, as they will often have a local mushroom grower, and supermarkets are now making lots of interesting varieties more readily available.

Preheat the oven to 140°C/fan 120°C/275°F/gas mark 1.

Clean the portobello mushrooms, peel them and remove the stalks, reserving the peelings and stalks. Put them, along with the shiitake mushrooms, in a deep ovenproof dish. Add the thyme, bay leaf, garlic, hot stock, wine, half the balsamic vinegar and dot 25g of the butter liberally over the top. Cover with foil and bake for 45 minutes.

Remove and leave to cool with the foil on. Strain the liquid through a muslin-lined sieve, reserving the shiitake and portobello mushrooms (discard the peel, stalks and herbs). This is your mushroom stock, the base of the soup.

Clean the rest of the mushrooms, quartering the chestnut mushrooms and tearing any oyster or girolles into pieces. Melt half the remaining butter in a large frying pan or wok, add the mushrooms and cook gently until soft, shaking the pan frequently. Pour in the remaining balsamic vinegar to deglaze the pan, then remove from the heat. Add the rest of the butter and set the pan aside. Season with salt and pepper. Heat the broth and taste it to check the seasoning, slice the reserved portobello and shiitake mushrooms and add them to the broth along with the rest of the mushrooms. Divide among serving bowls and eat immediately.

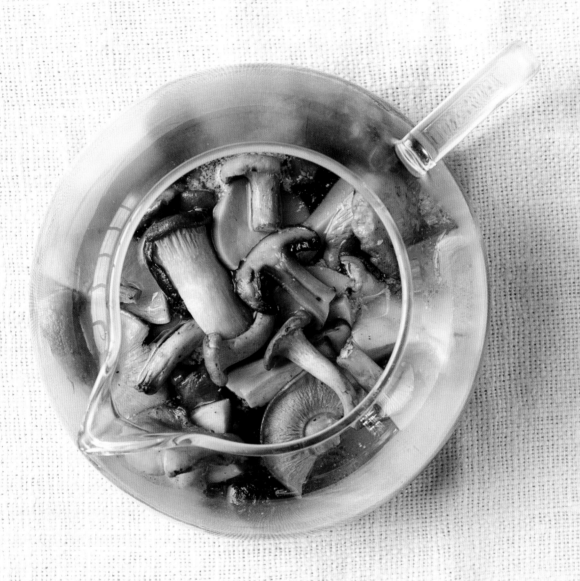

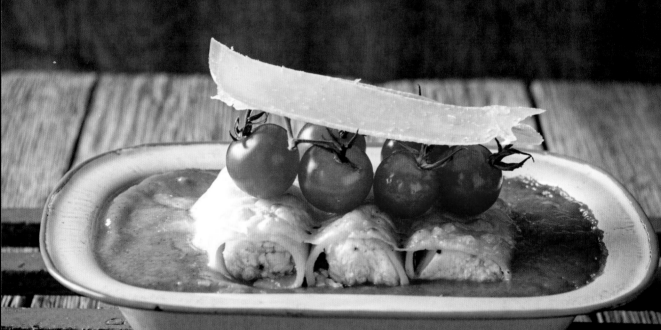

CINNAMON & PUMPKIN SOUP
WITH CANNELLONI

SERVES 4

750g peeled and cubed
   pumpkin or squash (about
   1kg unpeeled)
2 tbsp groundnut oil
2 tsp ground cinnamon
200g cherry tomatoes
2 tbsp balsamic vinegar
400ml hot vegetable stock
   (page 15)
6 dried cannelloni pasta shells
200g ricotta
1 tsp Chinese five-spice
zest of 1 lime, grated
Parmesan cheese, grated, plus
   a few shavings, to serve
flaky sea salt

This is almost a baked soup, which allows the pasta to be truly at one with the pumpkin. It's a warming, satisfying, autumn feast of a soup.

Preheat the oven to 220°C/fan 200°C/425°F/gas mark 7.

In a large bowl, mix the pumpkin with the oil and cinnamon. Place on a baking tray and roast for 30 minutes, or until cooked through and golden. Check halfway through and give the tray a shake. When the pumpkin pieces are cooked, place half the cherry tomatoes over the top and splash with the balsamic vinegar. Return to the oven, but turn it off; the residual heat will be enough to just burst the tomatoes after about 10 minutes.

Turn the oven down to 190°C/fan 170°C/375°F/gas mark 5.

Process the pumpkin and tomatoes in a blender until smooth, adding enough hot vegetable stock to reach the consistency you like (this soup is best quite thick). Taste and season with salt.

Meanwhile, mix the ricotta with the Chinese five-spice and lime zest and pipe the mixture into the centre of the cannelloni shells. Wrap each shell tightly in cling film. Bring a pan of water to the boil and gently lower in the cannelloni, then boil for 30 minutes. Allow to cool a little, then unwrap the cannelloni and cut them in half. Place each cannelloni half in the middle of an individual ovenproof dish and pour the soup around it. Top with Parmesan, then place in the oven for 20–25 minutes, or until bubbling at the edges. Place the reserved cherry tomatoes and Parmesan shavings on top and serve.

MARROW SOUP WITH COURGETTE FLOWERS & PESTO QUINOA

SERVES 4

2 medium marrows
2 tbsp groundnut oil
1 litre hot vegetable stock
    (page 15)
2 tbsp crème fraîche
1 tbsp miso glaze (or mix 1 tsp
    white miso paste with 1 tsp
    soft unsalted butter)
100g cooked quinoa
1 tbsp basil pesto
1 tbsp fresh tarragon, chopped
zest of 1 lime, grated
1 tbsp salted capers, rinsed,
    drained and chopped
1 tbsp grated Parmesan cheese
1 tsp unsalted butter
flaky sea salt and freshly
    ground black pepper
pumpkin seeds, to serve
thyme leaves, to serve

For the courgette flowers
    (optional)
300ml vegetable oil
8 courgette flowers
1 egg, beaten
1 tbsp cornflour

For Nicole, this is a pure taste of home: marrows are plentiful in Malta and marrow soup is revered. Combining the smooth soup with the roasted marrow and pesto quinoa turns this humble vegetable into a treat.

Top and tail the marrows and chop one of them into cubes. Heat the groundnut oil in a large frying pan, add the cubed marrow and cook gently until golden. Add the hot vegetable stock and simmer for about 10 minutes, or until the marrow is soft. Remove from the heat and process the marrow and stock in a blender until smooth. Stir in the crème fraîche, taste and season with salt.

Preheat the oven to 210°C/fan 190°C/410°F/gas mark 7. Slice the second marrow into 4 thick rings. Scoop out the inner flesh and brush each slice with miso glaze. Put the quinoa, pesto, tarragon, lime zest, capers and Parmesan in a bowl, mix well and season with sea salt and pepper.

Place the marrow slices on a baking tray and fill them with the quinoa mixture. Brush with butter and roast for about 20 minutes, or until the top of the marrow can easily be pierced with a fork. Remove the marrow slices and place in individual bowls. Pour the hot soup around the marrow.

For extra credit, serve with deep-fried courgette flowers. Heat the oil to 160°C/320°F. If you don't have a thermometer, you can test the oil by carefully dropping in a small cube of bread, which should bubble immediately; if it drops to the bottom, the oil isn't hot enough. Dip the courgette flowers in the egg and then the cornflour. Gently lower them into the oil with a slotted spoon and fry for about 5 minutes, or until crisp. Carefully remove them from the oil and drain on kitchen paper. Garnish the soup with the flowers, pumpkin seeds and thyme leaves and serve.

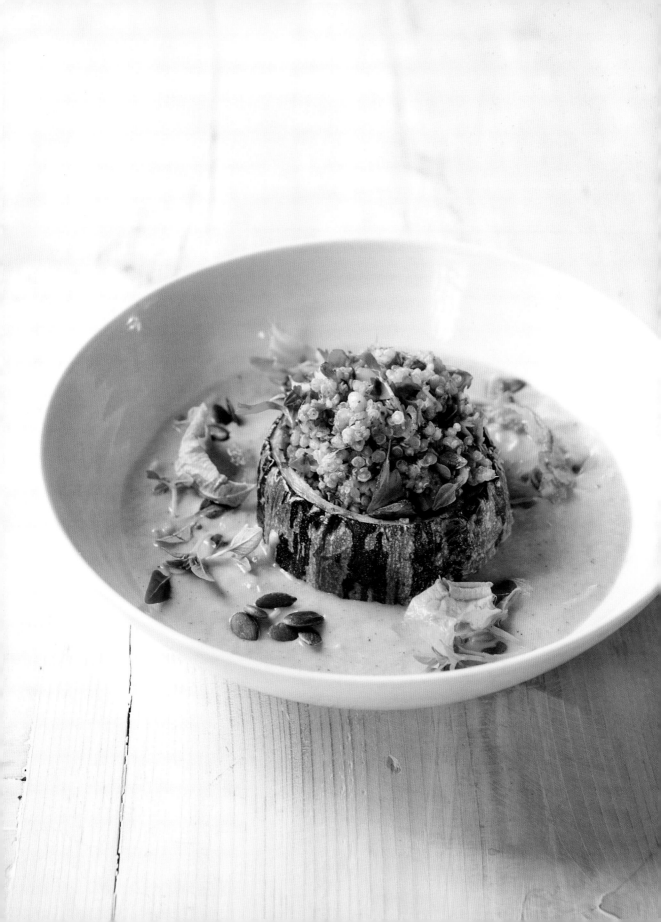

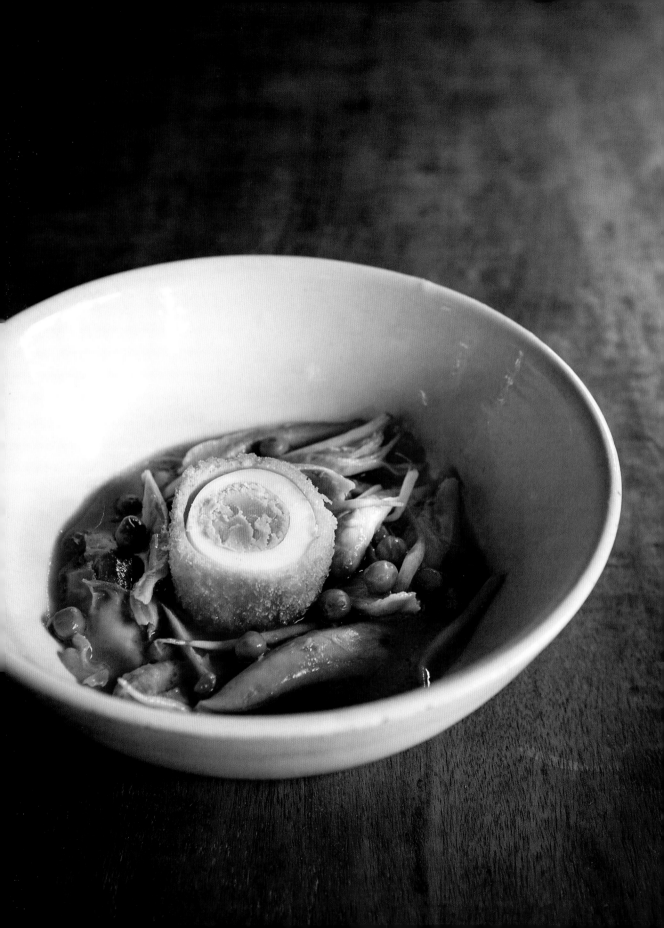

CHICKEN SOUP FOR THE SOUL

SERVES 2

4 chicken legs or 2 large
    chicken thighs, skin on and
    bone in
½ tsp ground turmeric
1 tsp fennel seeds
a pinch of chilli flakes
1 tbsp groundnut oil
olive oil, for frying
approximately 500ml hot
    chicken stock (page 14)
4 dried or fresh curry leaves
2 garlic cloves, bashed, with
    skin on
2 bay leaves
a few strips of unwaxed
    lemon zest
50g fresh peas
50g beansprouts

For the eggs
300ml vegetable oil
3 eggs
50g plain flour
70g panko breadcrumbs

Nicole loves this soup because it feels like a really satisfying meal, but in soup form. 'It's soul food, you know. When you read the ingredients you can feel the goodness. My mouth begins to water. Everything just seems to come together for this soup – every ingredient knows its place.'

In a large mixing bowl, toss the chicken pieces with the turmeric, fennel seeds, chilli flakes and groundnut oil. Leave to marinate for 30 minutes.

Heat the oil in a large pan, add the curry leaves and stir for a few seconds to infuse the oil. Remove the leaves with a slotted spoon. Add the chicken pieces to the pan and brown on all sides, then pour in the hot stock, garlic, curry leaves, bay leaves and lemon zest. Simmer gently for 45 minutes to 1 hour, or until the meat easily falls off the bone.

Meanwhile, boil 2 of the eggs for 6 minutes (start timing when you add the eggs to boiling water). Cool them under cold running water, then peel. Put the flour in a wide shallow bowl and season, beat the remaining egg in a second bowl, then tip the breadcrumbs into a third bowl.

Heat the oil to 160°C/320°F. If you don't have a thermometer, you can test the oil by carefully dropping in a small cube of bread, which should bubble immediately; if it drops to the bottom, the oil isn't hot enough. Dip each boiled egg in the flour, then the beaten egg, then the breadcrumbs. Gently lower them into the oil with a slotted spoon and fry for about 5 minutes, or until crispy. Carefully remove them from the oil and drain on kitchen paper.

Remove the chicken pieces from the soup and take the meat off the bones. Return the meat to the soup along with the peas and beansprouts. Divide the soup among the bowls and top with an egg.

A FEAST OF SEVEN FISH

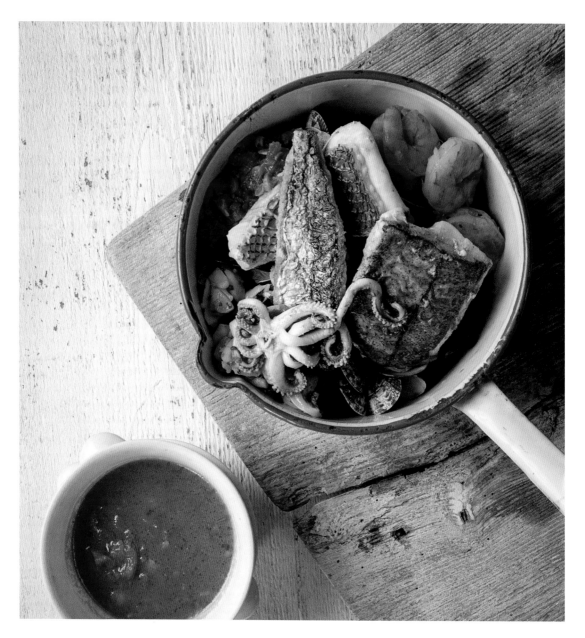

SERVES 4-6

200g ripe tomatoes

olive oil, for frying

1 onion, chopped

1 celery stalk, sliced

1 leek, sliced

2 garlic cloves, crushed

a pinch of saffron strands

a bouquet garni of bay and
    lemon thyme

1 tbsp sundried tomato paste

1.2 litres fish or vegetable stock
    (page 15)

about 1.5 kg mixed fresh fish
    fillets and cleaned shellfish
    (we used 1 large squid for
    calamari, 500g mussels,
    250g clams, 400g raw
    shelled prawns, 1 cod fillet,
    1 red snapper fillet and
    2 mackerel fillets, skin-on)

1 tsp fennel seeds

1/2 tsp dried chilli flakes

70g unsalted butter

2 spring onions, sliced

30ml vermouth or Nolly Prat

30ml single cream

1 tbsp salted capers, rinsed and
    drained

2 limes, to serve

flaky sea salt

Nicole put her heart and soul into preparing this soup for a grand feast to feed seven hungry women. It is based loosely on a traditional bouillabaisse, and it reminds us of the south of France, where a friend has a caravan that looks out over the hills leading down to the sparkling Mediterranean. Kate remembers family holidays in France where the main event was always the platter of *fruits de mer* from the van in the beach car park. All we'd add now is a glass or two of rosé.

Bring a pan of water to the boil and scald the tomatoes for 1 minute. Drain and refresh them in cold water then peel and chop them.

Heat the oil in a large, heavy-based pan, add the onion, about two thirds of the celery and leek and cook gently for about 10 minutes, until soft. Add the garlic and saffron strands, and after a couple of minutes, add the bouquet garni, chopped tomatoes, tomato paste and stock. Bring to the boil, then reduce to a simmer and cook over a low heat for 45 minutes. Taste for seasoning.

Meanwhile, prepare the fish. Rinse the squid and cut it so that it lies flat on the chopping board. Use a sharp knife to score the squid with a criss-cross pattern, then slice it into chunky calamari strips. Mix the calamari in a bowl with the fennel seeds and chilli flakes and set aside for a few minutes. Heat a dash of oil in a small pan over a low heat and cook the calamari for 1–2 minutes until they curl. Remove from the heat and set aside.

Melt half the butter in a large heavy-based pan, add the spring onions and remaining celery and leek and cook gently for about 15 minutes until soft. Add the mussels and clams, give the pan a good shake and cover with the lid until the shells begin to open. Discard any unopened shells. Pour in the vermouth and cream and simmer for 10 minutes. For the last 5 minutes, add the prawns and cook until they turn pink.

Preheat the oven to 190°C/fan 170°C/375°F/gas mark 5.

Meanwhile, cook the fish fillets. Heat a dash of oil in a non-stick pan. Season the cod and snapper fillets well and place skin-side down onto the pan. Once the skin is crispy, add the capers and a knob of butter to the pan and finish off the cooking in the oven for 5 minutes. Fry the mackerel fillets skin-side down in a little oil for 3 minutes, until the skin crisps. Flip it over and take the pan off the heat (the residual heat in the pan will be enough to finish cooking the fillets).

To serve, warm the saffron tomato broth and put in a large bowl. Place all the cooked fish and shellfish, along with the liquid from the shellfish, in a large serving bowl and squeeze over the lime. Grab some bowls and share among friends.

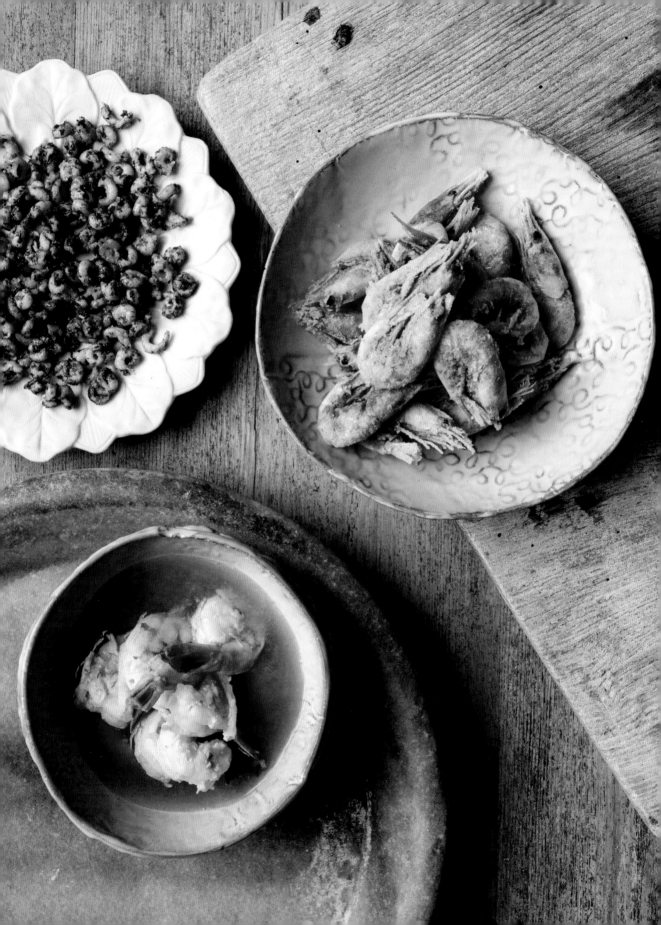

PRAWNS, PRAWNS, PRAWNS

SERVES 4

8 raw whole Atlantic prawns,
   with heads and shells
1 small piece fresh root ginger
   (about 2cm squared)
1 tbsp sweet chilli sauce
zest of a lime, finely grated
3 tbsp unsalted butter
3 tbsp nori flakes
100g cooked brown shrimp
200g soft-shell prawns
50g cornflour, mixed with 1 tsp
   chilli flakes
50ml vegetable oil

We use three types of prawns for this soup, which is a little extravagant, but each type adds its own flavours and textures. A real taste of the sea. If you can't find nori flakes, then 1 tablespoon lime zest or 2 tablespoons chopped capers will work nicely with this soup too. To make either of these flavoured butters, follow the same process as for the nori butter.

To make the stock for the soup, remove the heads and shells from the Atlantic prawns and place them in a pan. Cover the shells with 1 litre water and add the ginger, sweet chilli sauce and lime zest. Bring to the boil and simmer gently for 1 hour. Pass the stock through a sieve lined with a muslin cloth to remove the impurities.

Meanwhile, de-vein the Atlantic prawns. Use a small, sharp knife to make a shallow cut along the length of the black line on the back of the prawn, then lift it out using the tip of your knife. This is an important step because if the black line is not removed, it can give an unpleasant taste.

To make the nori butter, melt the butter in a pan and add the nori flakes. Transfer it to another receptacle and allow it to cool to room temperature.

Heat a ridged grill pan until very hot, add the Atlantic prawns and cook, turning them with tongs until just pink. Add the brown shrimp and then the nori butter. Remove the pan from the heat and once the butter has melted, spoon over the prawns.

Pat the soft-shell prawns in the spiced cornflour and shallow fry in vegetable oil until crispy. Remove and place on kitchen paper.

Divide all three types of prawns equally among bowls and ladle over the hot prawn broth.

MUSSELS & POLENTA

SERVES 4

400ml milk
2 garlic cloves, bashed
a bunch of fresh sage
2kg mussels, cleaned
1 tbsp light olive oil
1 onion, finely chopped
1 celery stalk, finely chopped
200ml dry cider
150g fine, quick-cook white or
    yellow polenta
20g grated Parmesan cheese
20g unsalted butter
flaky sea salt and freshly
    ground black pepper
croutons, to serve

Mussels are usually great value and excellent quality, and they aren't as tricky to prepare as you might think. When choosing them, do keep an eye out to make sure all the shells are closed and unbroken.

Pour the milk into a pan, bring to just below boiling point and add the garlic cloves and sage. Season with salt and pepper to taste. Remove from the heat, leave to cool and place in the refrigerator overnight to infuse.

Check through the mussels, discarding any open ones that don't close when tapped firmly on the work surface. Scrub off any barnacles if necessary.

Heat the oil in a heavy-based saucepan, add the onion and celery and cook gently until softened, then add the cider. Add the mussels to the pan, give them a good stir, cover with a lid and then remove the pan from the heat. Allow it to sit with the lid still on so the mussels cook in the residual heat. The mussels will open once cooked. Strain the contents of the pan over a bowl, reserving the liquid.

To make the polenta, bring the infused milk to the boil and stir in the polenta, whisking rapidly as you do so. You want it to be the consistency of a thick soup. Stir in the Parmesan and butter and taste for seasoning. Warm through the liquid reserved from the mussels. Divide the polenta among the serving bowls, top with the mussels and ladle the mussel broth over the top. Serve alongside a bowl of croutons.

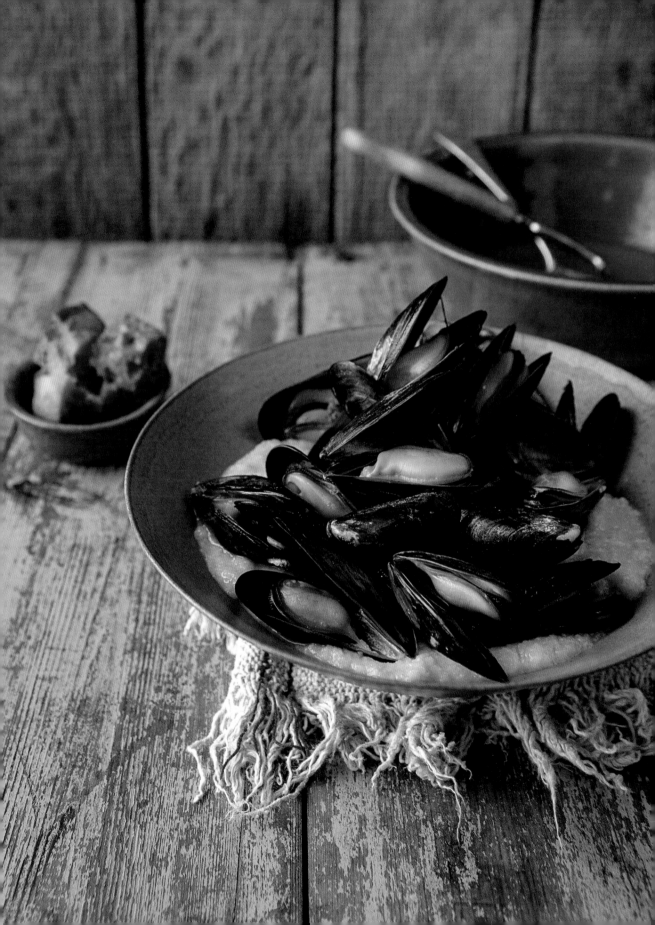

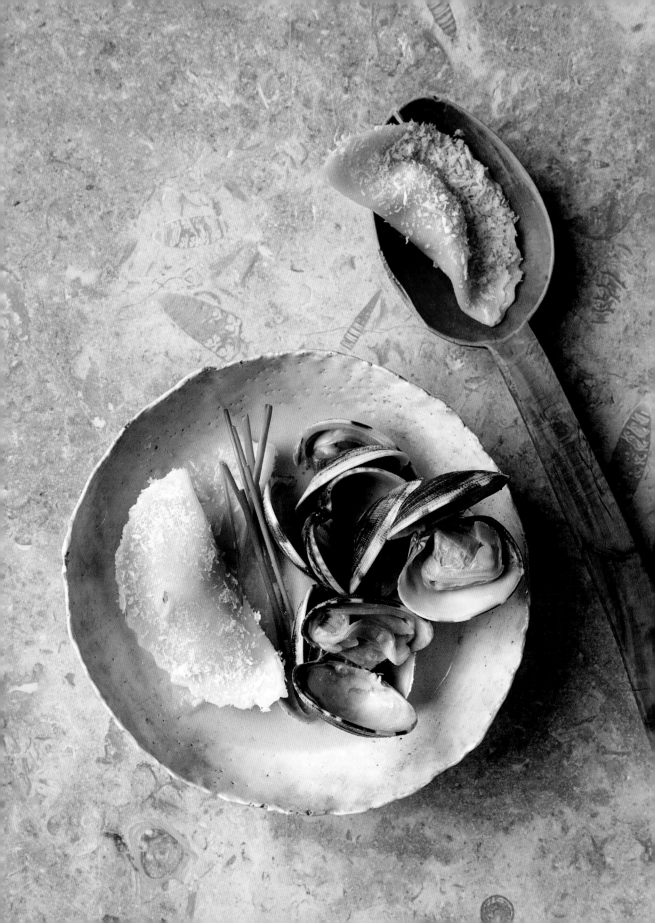

CLAMS & RAVIOLI

SERVES 2

20g unsalted butter

1 leek, white and pale green part only, thinly sliced

1 green chilli, thinly sliced

2cm piece fresh root ginger, finely chopped

500g fresh clams, cleaned and rinsed well to remove any grit

200ml sake

1 tsp sweet chilli sauce

500ml coconut milk drink (such as Alpro or Koko)

50ml fish sauce

3 pandan leaves, scrunched (optional)

fresh chives, chopped, to serve

For the crab ravioli

1 large sheet of fresh pasta

60g fresh white crabmeat

1 tbsp crème fraîche

1/2 red chilli, de-seeded and finely chopped

1 spring onion, finely chopped

egg yolk, lightly beaten

flaky sea salt and freshly ground black pepper

This soup brings shellfish and pasta together in happy union, but involves less pasta than our favourite, *spaghetti alle vongole*. Great for when you want to impress but still keep things on the lighter side.

First, make the crab ravioli (you'll need 3 per portion). Use a 8cm cookie cutter to cut out rounds from the pasta. Mix together all the remaining ingredients for the ravioli (except the egg yolk) and spoon a little into the centre of each of the pasta rounds. Brush egg yolk around the edges of the pasta, fold over to make a half-moon shapes and press the edges together well. To cook, bring a pan of water to the boil and add the ravioli. Simmer for 2 minutes, or until they float to the top of the water, before removing with a slotted spoon.

Melt the butter in a pan, add the leek, chilli and ginger and cook for a few minutes, until soft. Check over the clams and discard any that are not tightly closed. Add the clams to the pan and stir over the heat for a few minutes until they begin to open.

Add the sake, stirring well to dislodge any sediment on the bottom of the pan, and let simmer for a minute before adding the sweet chilli sauce, coconut milk drink, fish sauce and pandan leaves. Allow all the flavours to infuse for a couple of minutes, then take off the heat and cover. Strain the liquid through a sieve, reserving the liquid. At this point, discard any unopened shells. Return the clams along with the liquid, back to the clean pan. Add the cooked pasta and heat gently to warm everything through. Serve garnished with chopped chives.

OX CHEEK BROTH

SERVES 4

For the broth
3 veal bones
1 onion, quartered
1 leek, roughly chopped
1 celery stalk, roughly chopped
1 garlic clove
5 chicken wings
1 calf's foot
250ml Madeira
250ml port
5-6 shallots, halved and tied
    in muslin

For the ox cheek
flaky sea salt, for marinating
coconut sugar, for marinating
1 tbsp pickling spice mixture
    (we use one that contains
    yellow mustard seeds, black
    pepper, fennel, allspice, dill
    seeds, cloves, cinnamon,
    mace, bay and chilli)
2 ox cheeks, approximately
    250g each
1 tbsp groundnut oil
200g Swiss chard, shredded
unsalted butter, for cooking
mixed sorrel leaves, to serve
flaky sea salt and freshly
    ground black pepper

This soup is not for the faint of heart, but it's intensely nourishing. Mrs Beeton described ox cheek soup as a 'useful soup for benevolent purposes', perhaps because it was such a wholesome way of using up an undervalued piece of meat. It is very giving. If you can't find the ingredients for the broth, use a good-quality beef stock or demi-glace, add the Madeira and port, and follow the rest of the steps. Start this recipe two days before you want to serve it.

First, prepare the broth. Preheat the oven to 220°C/fan 200°C/425°F/gas mark 7. Put the veal bones in a large roasting tray and roast for 4-5 hours, until they are well browned. Transfer the bones to a large pot and cover with water. Add the onion, leek, celery and garlic and bring to the boil. Add the chicken wings and calf's foot, then reduce the heat to a simmer and cook gently over a very low heat for up to 8 hours.

To prepare the ox cheek, mix the dry brine mix of salt, coconut sugar and pickling spices and coat the ox cheek in the mixture. Leave it in the refrigerator overnight.

The next day, strain the broth through a muslin-lined sieve and discard the bones. Return the liquid to the heat and add the Madeira, port and shallots. Simmer gently to reduce it for 2-3 hours until thick and velvety in consistency.

Rinse the ox cheek and pat dry with kitchen paper. Preheat the oven to 150°C/fan 130°C/300°F/gas mark 2. Heat the oil in a heavy-based ovenproof casserole dish, add the ox cheek and brown it on both sides. Heat the broth and add it to the pan with the ox cheek, bring it to the boil, then cook in the oven for 4 hours, or until the meat is very tender. Taste for seasoning and allow it to cool in the oven overnight.

When you are ready to serve, rinse the Swiss chard and heat a hot wok with a little butter and a pinch of salt. Add the chard and cook until wilted (the water from rinsing is enough to steam them). Slice the ox cheek and heat through in the broth and then divide among bowls, with chard and sorrel leaves on the side ready to add just before eating.

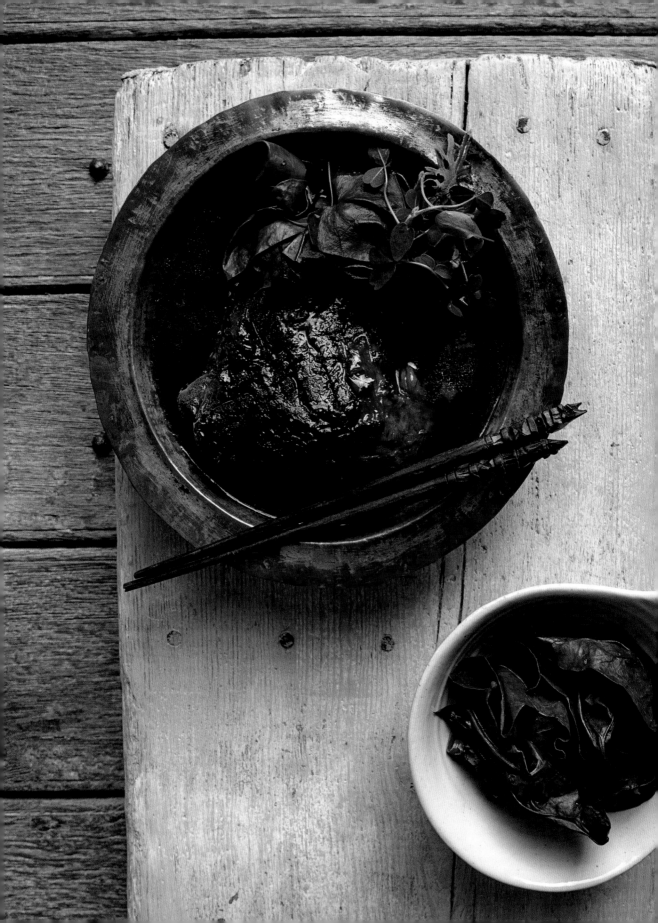

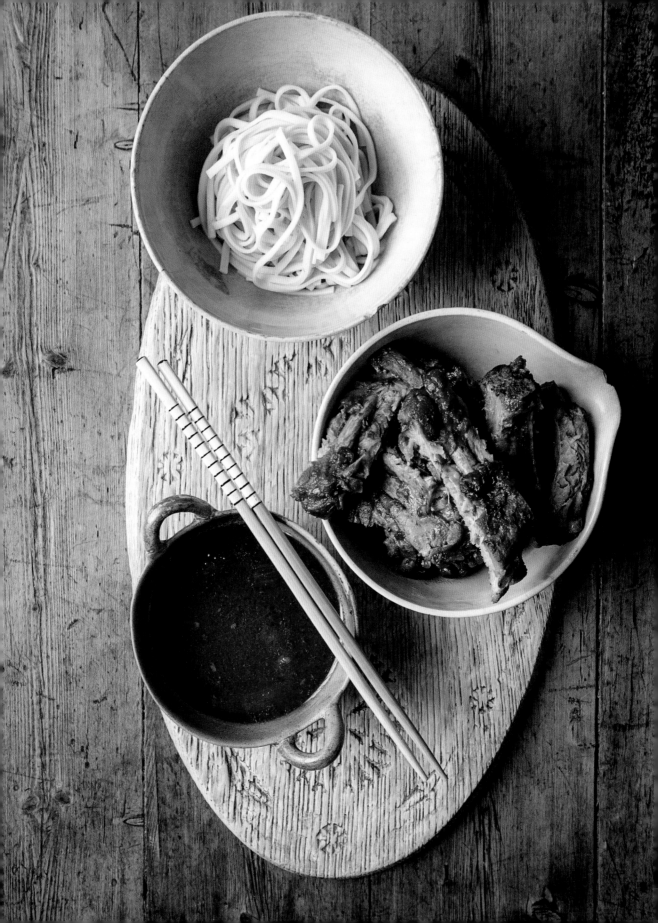

HOISIN RIBS WITH BROTH

SERVES 4

1 litre hot chicken stock
   (page 14)
250ml hoisin sauce
250ml freshly squeezed
   orange juice
10 pandan leaves (optional)
3 garlic cloves, crushed
a thumb-size piece of ginger,
   cut into 3 pieces
1 side of pork ribs, about
   800g–1kg
200g udon or rice noodles

Asian food in particular has inspired us to think of soups as feasts in their own right rather than just a quiet start to a meal. Ribs are often great value, so don't just wait until the summer barbecue season to enjoy them.

Preheat the oven to 170°C/fan 150°C/340°F/gas mark 3.

Put the stock, hoisin sauce and orange juice in a pan, bring to the boil and reduce the heat to a simmer. Layer the pandan leaves, if using, in a roasting tin and add the garlic and ginger, then place the pork ribs on top. Pour over the hoisin-orange sauce, cover with foil and roast for about 1 1/2 hours. Switch off the oven and leave to cool in the oven.

When ready to serve, remove the ribs and pour the liquid from the roasting dish into a pan. Bring to the boil and simmer for a few minutes. Meanwhile, cook the noodles in boiling water according to the packet instructions until tender. To serve, divide the noodles and pork ribs between bowls. Pour over the hot stock and enjoy.

BRAISED BEEF, HERITAGE RADISHES, BABY BEETS & HORSERADISH CREAM

SERVES 4

For the beef

1 tbsp white miso paste

1 tbsp Dijon mustard

500g beef brisket or beef shoulder steak

2 tbsp vegetable oil

4 shallots, peeled and halved

1 garlic clove, sliced

250ml good red wine

500ml beef or vegetable stock (pages 16 and 15)

1 tbsp tomato purée

2 bay leaves

1 tbsp date syrup

For the vegetables

500ml vegetable stock (page 15)

200g baby turnips, carrots and beetroot

200g mixed heritage radishes (or French Breakfast radishes)

1 Chinese cabbage, outer leaves removed and quartered

1 tbsp grated fresh horseradish (if available; jarred horseradish is also fine)

2 tbsp mascarpone

unsalted butter, to serve

We love Sundays and this tastes like Sunday in a bowl. Letting a simple cut of beef like brisket braise gently in some good red wine for a few hours makes it melt-in-the-mouth tender and deep with flavour.

Preheat the oven to 150°C/fan 130°C/300°F/gas mark 2.

Prepare the beef. Mix together the miso paste and Dijon mustard and roll the brisket in it. Chill in the fridge for a couple of hours or overnight.

Heat the oil until very hot in a large, heavy-based, ovenproof casserole, add the beef and cook briefly to sear on both sides. Remove the beef and set aside, then add the shallots to the dish and brown for a few minutes. Return the beef to the pan, along with the the rest of the ingredients, and scrape the base of the pan with a wooden spoon or spatula to loosen the caramelised bits at the bottom. Bring to a simmer, then take off the heat. Put the lid on and transfer to the oven to stew for 5–6 hours, until the beef is tender. Allow to cool and leave to rest for 1 hour.

For the vegetables, bring the stock to the boil in a large, shallow pan. Add the baby vegetables, then cover and simmer over a very low heat until almost tender. (Cooking the vegetables on a very low heat will mean they keep their shape and colour.) Add the radishes and Chinese cabbage for the last 3 minutes.

Meanwhile, mix the horseradish with the mascarpone. Add it a little at a time and keep tasting until it's hot enough for you.

To serve, remove the beef from the broth and set aside. Bring the broth to a simmer and allow it to reduce, skimming off any impurities. When you are happy with the flavour and consistency of your broth, pull the beef apart and warm it through, then take 4 serving bowls and divide the beef between them, adding a small knob of butter to each bowl. Next, divide the vegetables among the bowls. Pour the hot soup slowly into the bowls. Serve with the horseradish mascarpone on the side.

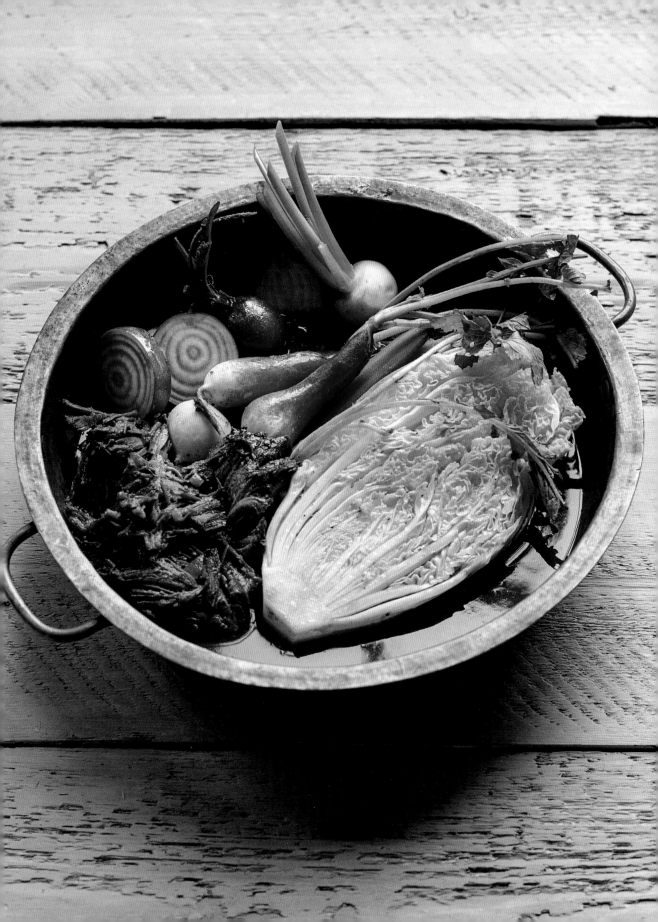

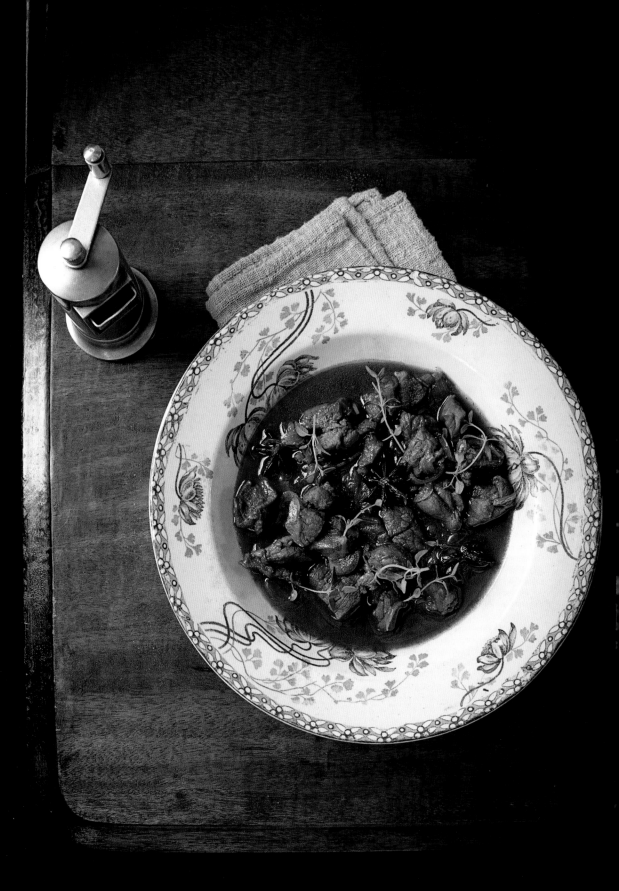

THIT HEO KHO

SERVES 4

vegetable oil, for frying
800g pork neck or shoulder,
    cut into 2cm cubes
4 shallots, chopped
2 garlic cloves, chopped
1 tbsp Chinese five-spice
6 star anise pods
125ml ponzu or tamari (soy)
    sauce
40g palm sugar, grated
40g coconut sugar or
    raw cane sugar
4 tbsp fish sauce
fresh thyme or coriander
    leaves, to garnish

Thit Heo Kho is a Vietnamese dish that is traditionally served with hard-boiled eggs. This is our version of Anna Hansen's Modern Pantry recipe for the dish. Pork is often very lean, but for this recipe you need a bit of fat, so ask for pork neck or shoulder, as these cuts are best for braising. Ponzu is a light soy sauce with a hint of citrus and is a great addition to your storecupboard (page 11). Any leftovers will be delicious, and you can bulk it up by adding some cooked pearl barley and some greens.

Preheat the oven to 140°C/fan 120°C/275°F/gas mark 1. Heat a little oil in a deep frying pan, add the pork in small batches and brown it on all sides. Lift out and set the pork aside.

Heat a little more oil in the pan, add the shallots and garlic, and cook until translucent. After 5 minutes, add the Chinese five-spice and continue to cook for another few minutes. Add the pork to the pan and stir everything thoroughly so that the pork is coated with the spices. Add 500ml water and all the remaining ingredients except the fresh herbs. Bring to a simmer, then cover with a lid and braise in the oven for about 1 hour, or until the pork is lovely and tender. Serve in bowls with fresh thyme or coriander leaves to garnish.

ASK YOUR BUTCHER

A friend of Nicole's did a *stage* (an unpaid restaurant work-experience placement) at Noma, one of the world's top restaurants, in Copenhagen. He said that the chefs got to know the cow they would use for carpaccio for around a year before it was slaughtered, and that it had the most perfect marbling. That may be a little extreme for most of us, but we're often so detached from our food these days as we choose from plastic-wrapped pieces of meat that seem a million miles away from the animal that was raised to produce it. Going to a good butcher, where you can see the meat up close and personal before you choose your cut, takes us a step closer. With a cut like rib-eye, you want to look for that marbling that Nicole's friend talked about. These soft lines of fat are what will give the meat fuller flavour.

Generally, beef should be a rich, velvety, deep red colour, and butchers will nearly always be happy to recommend a cut or give a little cooking advice. They will often be able to source unusual cuts, such as ox cheek (page 188) or marrow bones (Nicole's favourite thing in the world), and also the cheaper cuts that work so well in soups and stews, such as brisket and shin. We often brine cuts of meat that contain a mixture of muscle, fat and connective tissue, such as beef shin, ox cheek or pork belly. This begins to break down the fat without tightening up the muscles, so that you can cook over a low heat for tenderness.

The provenance of food is something that we try to understand as much as we can. The more information a butcher or greengrocer can give us about where their produce comes from the better, because it will tend to indicate high ethical standards. It's not always easy to determine, but grass-fed beef is our preferred choice. We tend to imagine all beef cattle grazing on rolling pastures, which is what they evolved to do, but most are fed on grain after six months to make them grow faster. Cows aren't designed to eat corn or other types of grain, so they will often be routinely given antibiotics to combat any problems with their digestion. An organic label doesn't guarantee better flavour, but we do go for the organic option because of the rigorous standards that have to be met for organic certification. The animals are required to be free range, must have access to fields when weather permits and have a certain amount of space to help reduce stress and disease. They are fed as natural a diet as possible, and are only given drugs to treat an illness; they also cannot be given growth hormones.

We tend to eat less meat (and fish, too), but spend a little more on quality and animal welfare. Living in the city, it isn't always easy to remember and respect where our food comes from, which is probably why we seek out farm shops and markets, whether at home or on our travels. Meeting the people who cultivate the soil, raise the animals or butcher the whole carcass helps us to realise the true value of food.

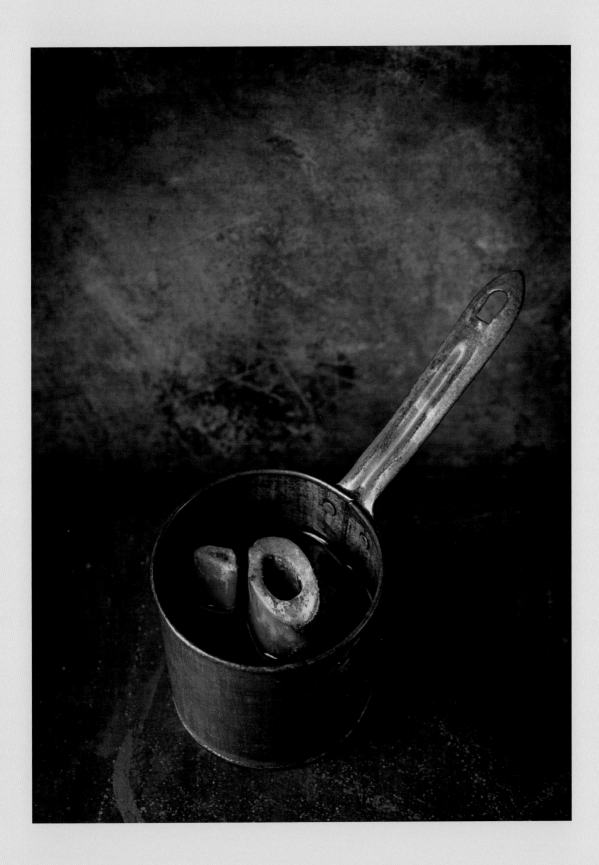

BAY LEAF BROTH
WITH VENISON MEATBALLS

SERVES 4

groundnut or olive oil, for frying
1 celery stalk, finely chopped
2 banana shallots, thinly sliced
1 tsp harissa paste
1 tsp tomato purée
200g egg or udon noodles,
   to serve

For the bay leaf broth

1 onion, halved
2 garlic cloves, bashed, with
   skin on
1 celery stalk, roughly chopped
1 whole red or green chilli
12 bay leaves, preferably fresh
a handful of fresh sage

For the meatballs

400g venison mince
1 onion, finely chopped
1 garlic clove, finely chopped
1 celery stalk, finely chopped
1 tsp mustard powder
1 vegetable stock cube,
   crumbled (or 1 tsp vegetable
   bouillon powder)
1 tsp tomato purée
1 tsp freshly grated horseradish
   (or 1 tsp hot horseradish
   cream)
1 egg, lightly beaten

This soup will keep you warm in the colder months. Venison is an excellent meat to try, if you haven't already: it's really tasty and also quite lean. The idea for the broth came from Kate's parents' garden, where a bay tree happily grows like mad. We get to dry huge bunches, ready to use in as many soups, stocks and stews as we can make.

Put the bay leaf broth ingredients in a large pan, cover with 1 litre water, bring to the boil and simmer for 2 hours. Pass through a sieve, reserving the liquid and bay leaves.

To make the meatballs, mix the ingredients well in a large bowl and divide the mixture into 8 meatballs, rolling it between your hands.

To make the soup, heat the oil in a large pan, add the meatballs and brown on all sides, then remove and set them aside. Add the celery and shallots and cook until soft.

Add the bay leaf broth and reserved bay leaves, bring to the boil and reduce the heat to a simmer. Add the harissa paste and tomato purée, then the meatballs. Simmer for 10–15 minutes. Meanwhile, cook the noodles according to the packet instructions. Divide among the bowls, top with the meatballs and pour over the bay leaf broth.

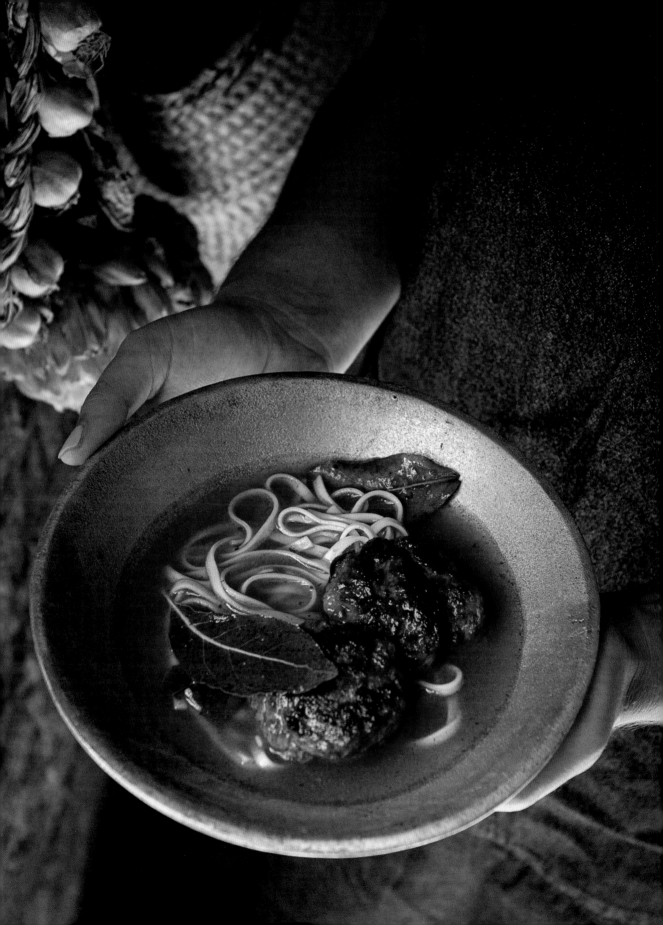

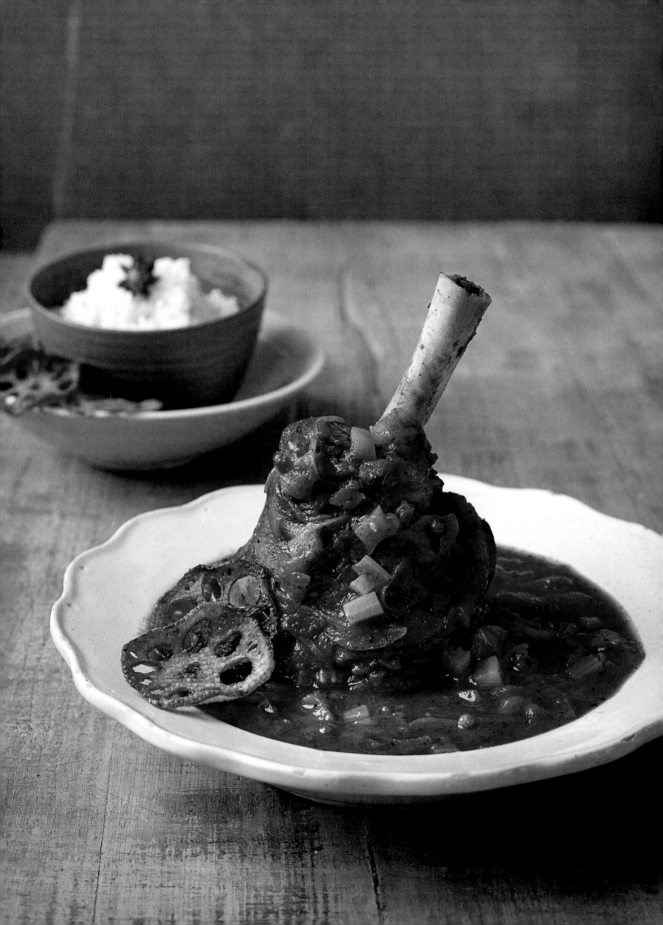

LAMB SHANK

SERVES 2

For the lamb

1 tbsp fennel seeds
1 tbsp juniper berries
1 tbsp black peppercorns
25g coconut or brown sugar
25g flaky sea salt
1 lamb shank (or 2 if you are
    very hungry)

For the soup

1 tbsp groundnut oil
30ml red wine
knob unsalted butter
1 onion, finely chopped
1 carrot, finely chopped
1 celery stalk, finely chopped
1 x 400g tin tomatoes
½ tbsp mango chutney
½ tbsp other chutney, such as
    apple and tomato
lotus root crisps (available from
    Asian stores), or 1 apple plus
    1 tbsp icing sugar, to serve
    (optional)
boiled rice, to serve

This soup is sweet, succulent and comforting. The lamb can take all the robust flavours of the spices and chutney, and melts in the mouth when cooked slowly and with patience. You can be safe in the knowledge that it will be worth it.

Grind the fennel seeds, juniper berries and black peppercorns in a spice grinder or pestle and mortar. Set half aside and mix the rest of it with the sugar and salt. Cover the lamb shank with the mixture and leave to brine in the refrigerator overnight.

The next day, preheat the oven to 150°C/fan 130°C/300°F/gas mark 2. Rinse the lamb to remove the brine. Heat the groundnut oil in a large ovenproof pan and once very hot, brown the lamb shank on all sides, then remove and set aside. Add the red wine to the pan and let it bubble, stirring to dissolve any sediment. Remove and set aside.

In the same pan, melt the butter, add the onion, carrot and celery and cook gently until soft. Make a bit of space in the pan and add the remaining spice mixture. Once the aromas begin to be released after a couple of minutes, stir the spices into the vegetables. Add the tomatoes, 200ml water, the chutneys and bring almost to the boil. Add the lamb shank and scrape the reserved juices into the pan. Cover and cook in the oven for 2 hours, or until the meat is very tender.

To make apple crisps, if using, thinly slice the apple into rings (a mandoline is ideal for this). Spread them out evenly on an oven tray and sprinkle with icing sugar. Bake in the oven until crisp, checking frequently.

Serve the lamb shank surrounded by sauce, with the lotus root or apple crisps to garnish (if using) and boiled rice on the side.

TURKEY, CRANBERRY & BRUSSELS SPROUTS

SERVES 4

For the turkey stock
leftover turkey bones
1 onion, halved
1 celery stalk
1 garlic clove, bashed
1 tbsp black or pink
    peppercorns
2 bay leaves

For the soup
40g unsalted butter
2 leeks, sliced
1 litre turkey stock (see above)
    or chicken stock (page 14)
200g turkey trimmings
200ml single cream
100g Brussels sprouts, thinly
    sliced
30g pine nuts
200g leftover turkey breast
    meat slices, cut into 1cm
    thick slices
50g dried cranberries, soaked
    in water or cranberry juice
flaky sea salt and freshly
    ground black pepper

After your Christmas dinner, save the turkey bones and carcass and then show your leftover turkey some love with the classic flavours of chestnut and Brussels sprouts.

Add all the stock ingredients to a large saucepan and cover with plenty of water. Bring to the boil and then simmer on a low heat for 2–3 hours until reduced down to about 1 litre. Strain the stock through a sieve and set aside. Pull off any meat from the bones and set aside also.

To make the soup, melt half the butter in a large saucepan and sauté the leek for 10–15 minutes until soft. Add the stock and turkey trimmings and bring to the boil. Reduce the heat, add the cream and simmer for 25–30 minutes. Process in a blender until smooth and taste for seasoning. If you prefer, pass the soup through a sieve.

Melt the remaining butter in a medium pan and sauté the sprouts. Season with a little salt and pepper. Toast the pine nuts in a dry pan until lightly golden.

To serve, ladle the hot soup into bowls, add the turkey slices and scatter over the cranberries, sprouts and pine nuts.

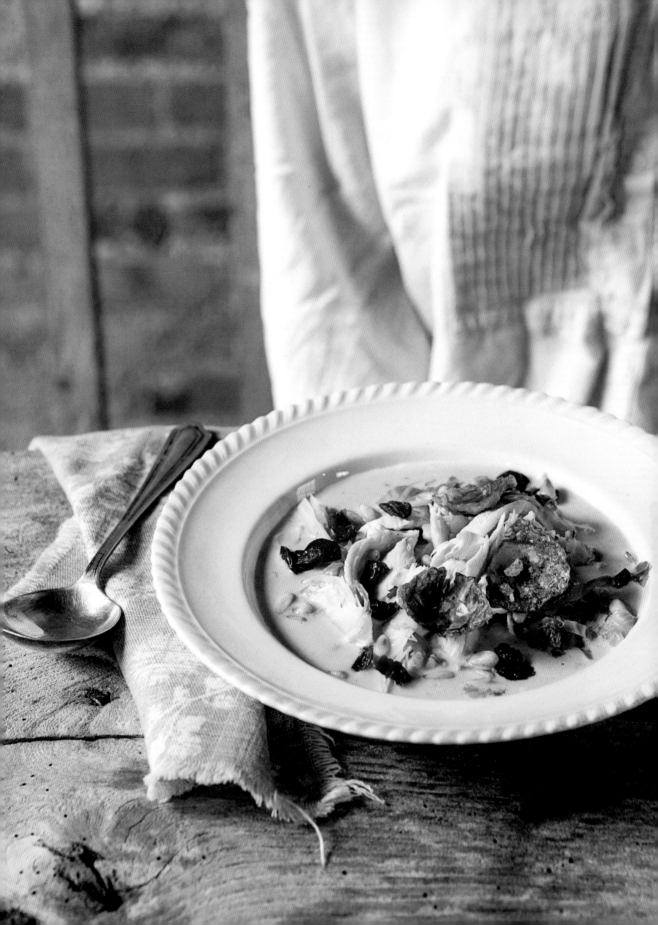

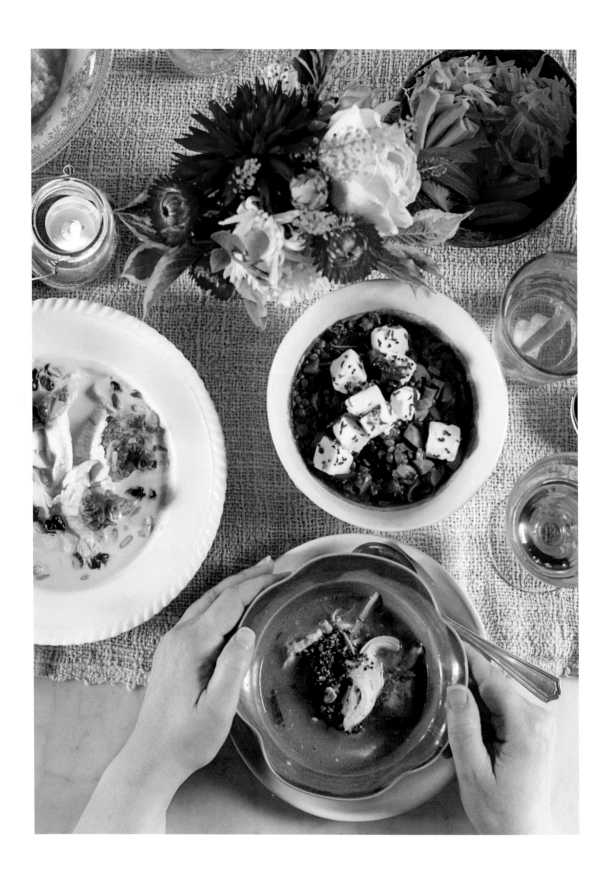

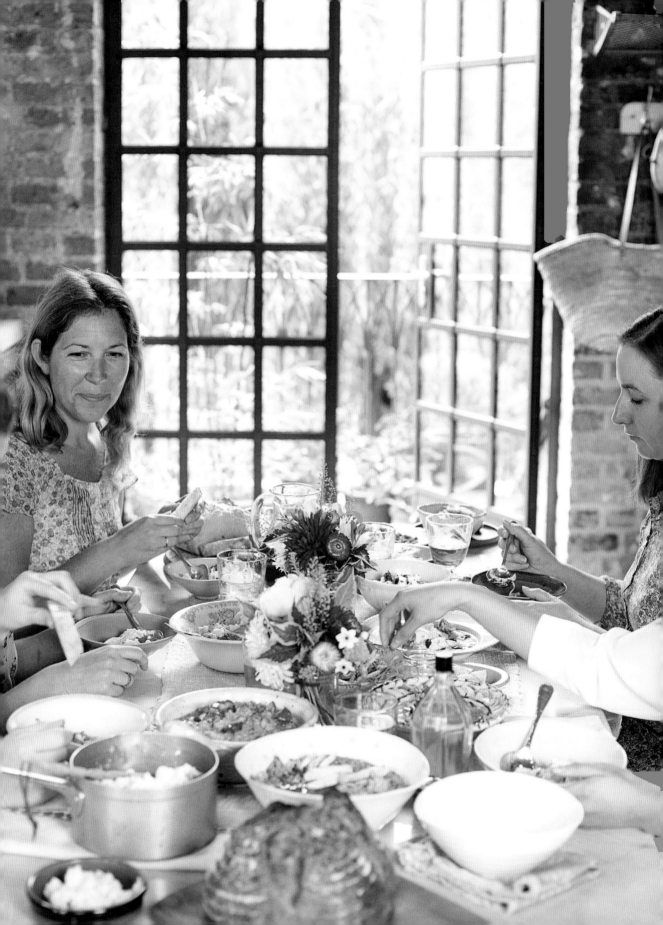

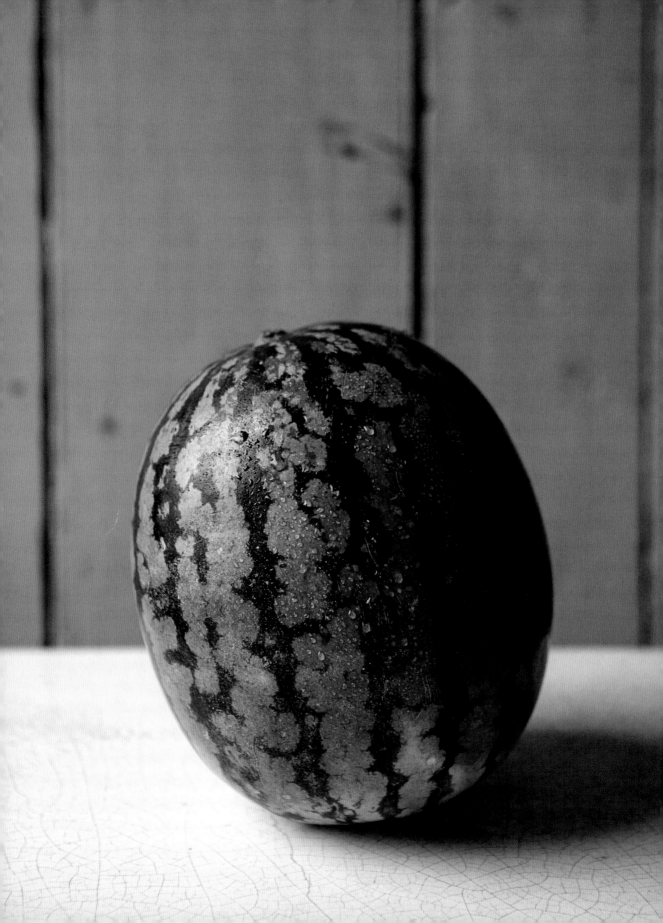

CHILLED

The clean flavours in cold soups come through simply and beautifully

You need a hot summer's night or day to go with it, but when there's warmth in the air and you can eat outside, a chilled soup such as Gazpacho or Vichyssoise is exactly the right choice. Not surprisingly, there's not much of a tradition of cold soups in northern Europe, but once you hit the south of France things start to make sense. The moment you try one for the first time you'll begin to realise what you've been missing out on.

Like many of the soups in this book, chilled soups work best with good-quality, seasonal ingredients, hence the cucumber, white asparagus, fennel and watermelon. Depending on your mood and the weather, quite a few soups from other chapters can be enjoyed cold, too, such as Good Woman's Soup or Celery Soup with Beetroot-cured Salmon. The trick with most chilled soups is to ensure they are very smooth, so passing them through a sieve before chilling will elevate them to the next level. We prefer our chilled soups not to be ice cold, so that we can taste the ingredients, and the clean flavours of fennel, asparagus or watermelon come through simply and beautifully.

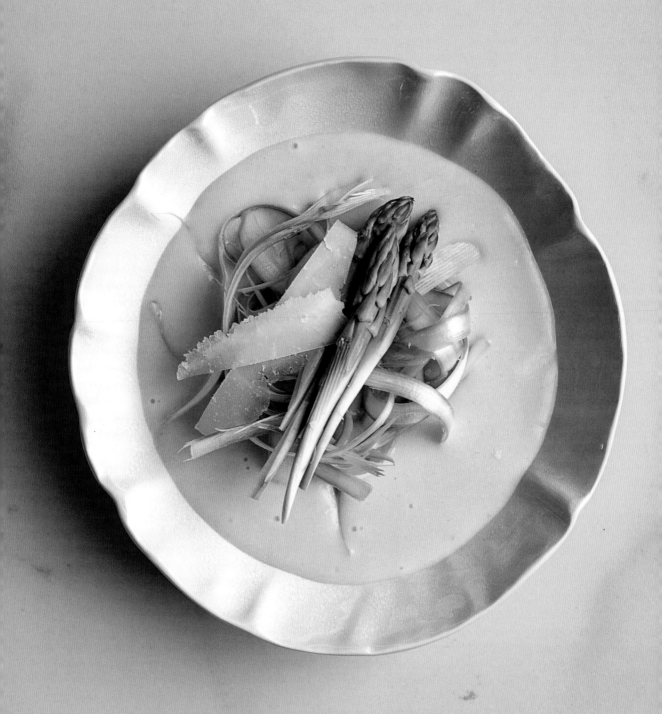

WHITE ASPARAGUS SOUP WITH SHAVED ASPARAGUS & PECORINO

SERVES 2

250g white asparagus
1 tbsp unsalted butter
about 600ml hot chicken stock
   (page 14)
1 tbsp mascarpone
a handful of green asparagus
flaky sea salt and freshly
   ground black pepper
6-8 green asparagus, to serve
pecorino cheese, to serve

White and purple asparagus is only around for a short time in spring, but do treat yourself if you spot it. This soup works just as well with green asparagus, but there's something quite astonishing about the flavour of white asparagus. There's hardly anything to do when making this soup; the ingredients sing for themselves. This soup is particularly good served chilled but also works well warm.

Snap off and discard the woody parts of the white asparagus and chop into 2.5cm pieces. Melt the butter in a pan, add the asparagus and sauté for 2 minutes before adding enough stock to cover.

Bring to the boil, then reduce the heat to a simmer and cook until the asparagus are tender, which will be slightly different each time but should only take a few minutes.

Process in a blender until smooth. Add the mascarpone, taste and season with salt and pepper and process again. Chill in the refrigerator for at least 2 hours before serving. Divide between 2 serving bowls. Use a vegetable peeler to create shavings of raw green asparagus and pecorino cheese and scatter them on top to serve.

CUCUMBER GAZPACHO

SERVES 2

1 cucumber, de-seeded and
  chopped (preferably the
  small Lebanese type, which
  doesn't need peeling; if using
  an ordinary variety, peel it)
1 slice stale sourdough bread
25g whole almonds, roasted
500ml unsweetened almond
  milk
1 tbsp extra-virgin olive oil
1 tbsp white balsamic vinegar
a handful of fresh mint
a handful of baby spinach
flaky sea salt and freshly
  ground black pepper

**For the seafood salad
  (optional)**
150g cooked white crabmeat
140g cooked crayfish tails
10g chives, finely chopped

Nicole loves 'clean' food: food that speaks for itself and doesn't confuse your tastebuds, but simply makes them happy. On a hot summer's day the cooling cucumber and mint are the perfect complement to a blue sky. We like to serve it with an assembled salad of crayfish and crabmeat.

Soak the cucumber, bread and almonds in the almond milk, oil and balsamic vinegar and leave in the refrigerator overnight. Before serving, process in a blender until smooth.

Add the mint and spinach and process again to give the soup a fresh green colour. Taste and season with salt and pepper.

To assemble the seafood salad, divide the crabmeat and crayfish tails into 2 glass bowls and top with a layer of chopped chives. Season with a salt and pepper and serve alongside the cucumber gazpacho.

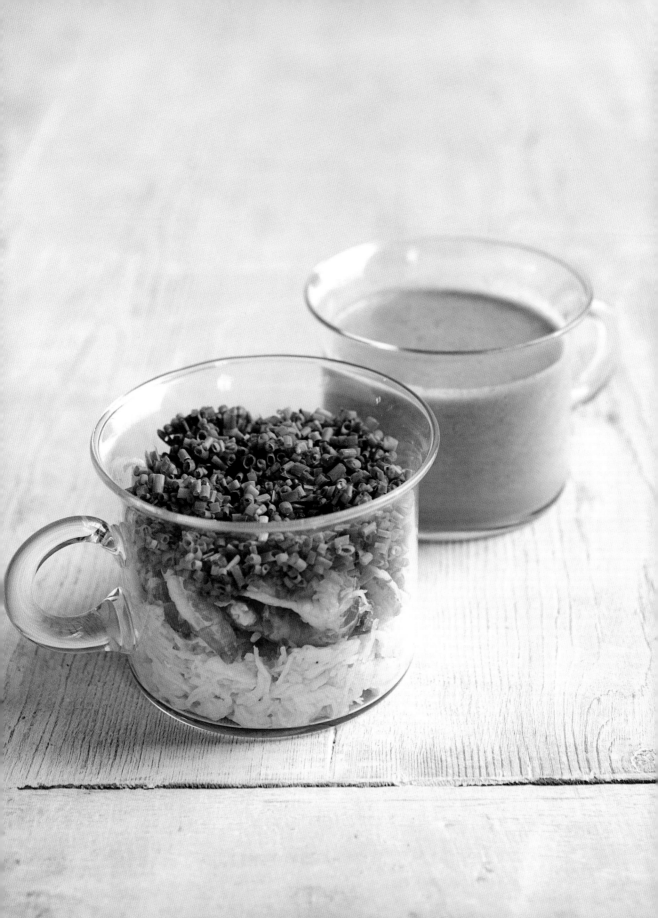

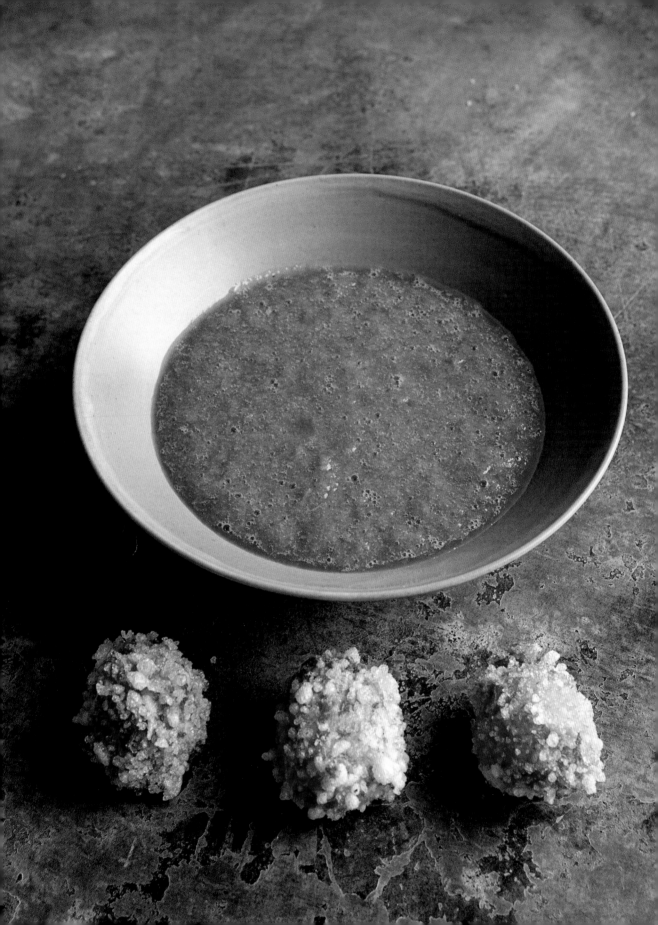

FENNEL VICHYSSOISE

SERVES 4

1 large fennel bulb or 2 smaller
    ones, sliced 5mm thick
2 tbsp sherry vinegar
800ml–1 litre vegetable or
    chicken stock (pages 14–15)
1 tbsp unsalted butter
1 medium leek or 2 small ones,
    finely sliced
1 large potato or 2 medium
    ones, approximately 300g,
    cut into 2cm cubes
100g baby spinach
flaky sea salt

For the quail eggs (optional)
300ml vegetable oil
4 hard-boiled and peeled
    quail eggs
50g plain flour
1 egg, lightly beaten
70g panko breadcrumbs

This soup really benefits from using homemade stock; it raises it to the level of oohs and aahs. Roasting the fennel with a little sherry vinegar encourages it to soften while caramelising it slightly, and works well whether you are making soup or serving it as a side. These quail eggs aren't essential, but they are delicious and just seem to work perfectly. This soup is also very good served hot, in which case you don't need to be so pernickety about sieving it.

Preheat the oven to 140°C/fan 120°C/285°F/gas mark 1.

In a bowl, toss the fennel with the sherry vinegar, season with salt and place in an oven dish. Add a splash of stock and cover tightly with kitchen foil. Roast in the oven for about 45 minutes, or until soft.

Meanwhile, melt the butter in a heavy-based saucepan, add the leek and cook gently for about 10 minutes, or until soft. Add the potatoes and continue to cook for 2 minutes, then add the remaining stock. Bring to the boil and simmer on a low heat for 10–15 minutes or until the potatoes are lightly cooked and easy to pierce with a sharp knife. Remove from the heat and process in a food processor until smooth, in batches if necessary, along with the roast fennel and handfuls of raw spinach, which give it a lovely colour. Pass the soup through a fine sieve to remove any stringy bits from the fennel and leek. You'll need to use the back of the ladle to really push it through. It takes a bit of time, but this gives you a beautifully smooth soup. Chill in the refrigerator until ready to serve.

For the quail eggs, heat the oil to 160°C/320°F. Dip each boiled egg in the flour, then the beaten egg, then the breadcrumbs. Gently lower them into the oil with a slotted spoon and fry for about 3 minutes, or until crispy. Carefully remove them from the oil and drain on kitchen paper. Serve each bowl of soup with a quail egg.

WATERMELON GAZPACHO

SERVES 4 AS A STARTER

1 tbsp olive oil

1 red bell pepper, sliced

1 shallot, sliced

750g watermelon, chopped
and de-seeded

500ml tomato juice

5 drops Tabasco

1 tsp Worcestershire sauce

1 tsp balsamic vinegar

1 passion fruit, juice and seeds
scooped out

flaky sea salt and freshly
ground black pepper

Our friend Sebastian is head chef at the Bella Luce Hotel in Guernsey, and introduced us to this wonderful watermelon gazpacho. It's lighter on tomato than many gazpacho recipes, and the perfect start to a Sunday lunch at the height of summer. If you're tempted to leave out the passion fruit, Nicole encourages you above all other tips in this book to include it! It changes everything.

Heat the olive oil in a pan, add the pepper and shallot and cook gently until soft. Put the watermelon in a blender along with the tomato juice and blend to a purée. Add all the other ingredients, season with salt and pepper and blend to a smooth consistency. Chill well before serving.

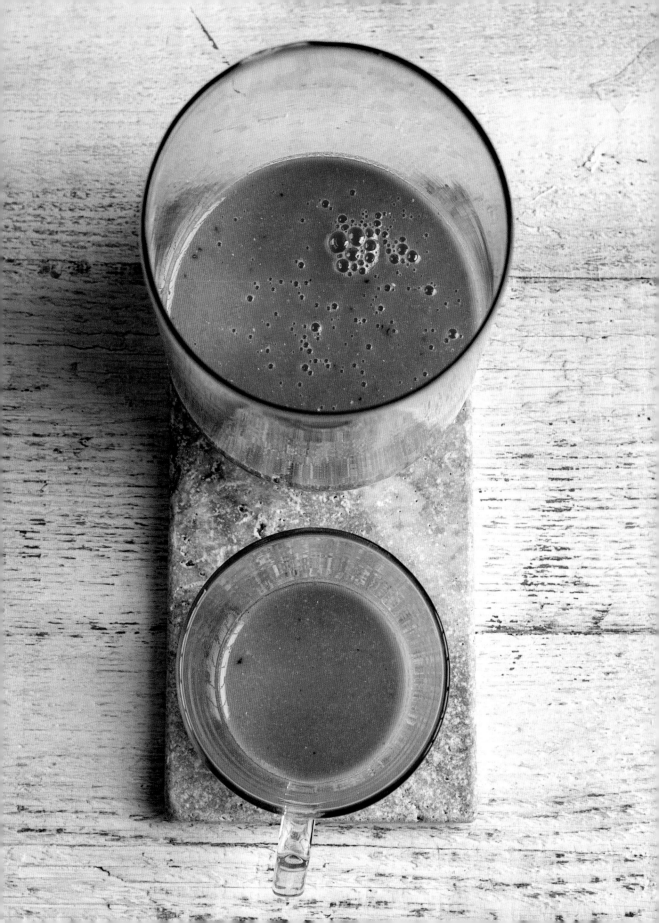

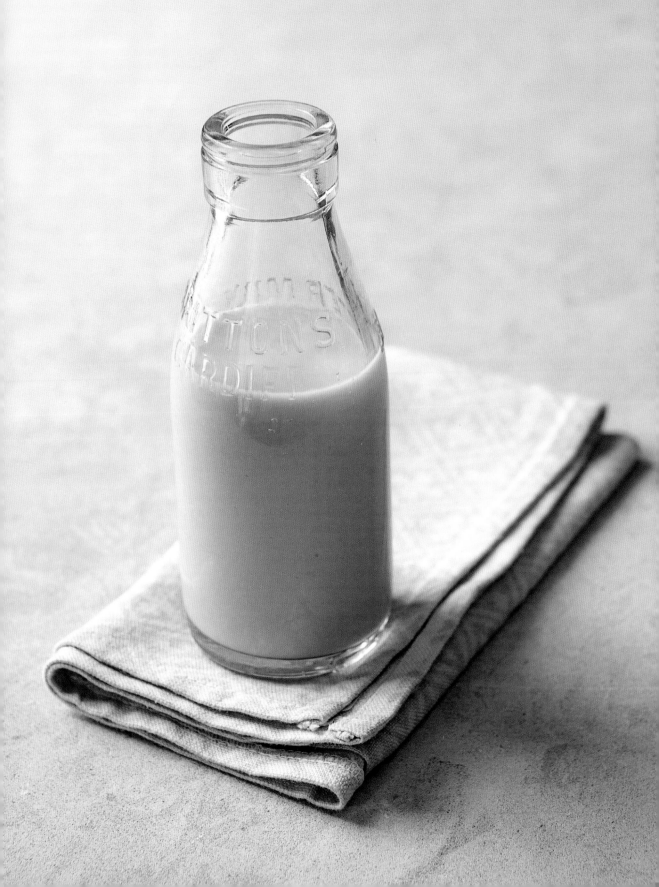

AVOCADO & RAW MILK

SERVES 4

2 large ripe Hass avocados
400ml raw milk (or use
    ordinary whole milk,
    or coconut milk drink such
    as Alpro or Koko)
1 tsp flaky sea salt
4 pinches cayenne pepper
juice of 2 limes

There is little more satisfying on a hot summer day than a perfectly ripe avocado. Raw (unpasteurised) milk is milk in its purest state, and is packed with flavour and beneficial bacteria. Some farmers are now certified to sell it here in the UK, and it can be found online and sometimes at farmers' markets.

Scoop out the flesh of the avocados into a blender with half the milk and process until smooth. Add the rest of the milk in stages until you reach your preferred consistency.

Add the salt, cayenne pepper and lime juice and blend again. Taste to check the flavour, and once you are happy, with it, pour the soup into container. Cover the top of the soup with cling film, pressing it down gently to touch the surface of the soup so that any air is excluded (this reduces the chance of the surface discolouring). Chill in the refrigerator, ideally for 6 hours and serve the soup in chilled glass milk bottles or tumblers.

WHITE ALMOND

SERVES 4

150g day-old, good-quality
white bread, crusts removed
100g blanched almonds
300ml milk
½ garlic clove, crushed
50ml olive oil
2 tbsp white balsamic vinegar
flaky sea salt
fried enoki mushrooms and
pancetta, to serve (optional)

This is inspired by a Greg Malouf recipe. Traditionally in Andalusia, white almond soup is served with grapes but we've substituted a few enoki mushrooms and crispy pancetta.

Put the bread and almonds in a bowl with the milk and garlic, cover and place in the refrigerator overnight.

The next day, place the bread mixture in a food processor. Process, adding the olive oil very slowly, then add 500ml iced water a little more quickly until the soup reaches the consistency of single cream. Add the vinegar and season with salt to taste. Serve chilled with a garnish of fried enoki mushrooms and pancetta, if you like.

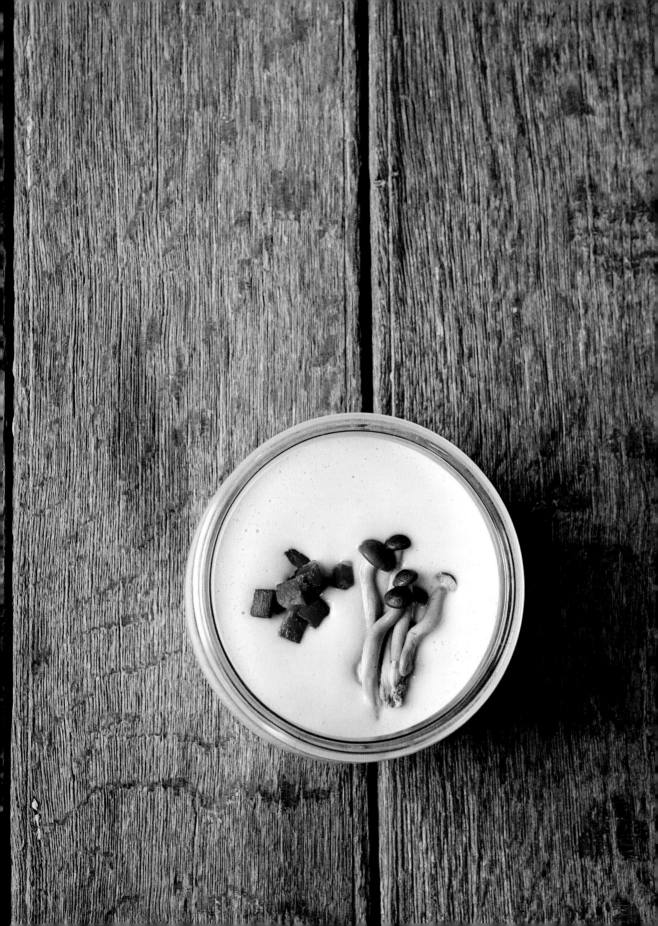

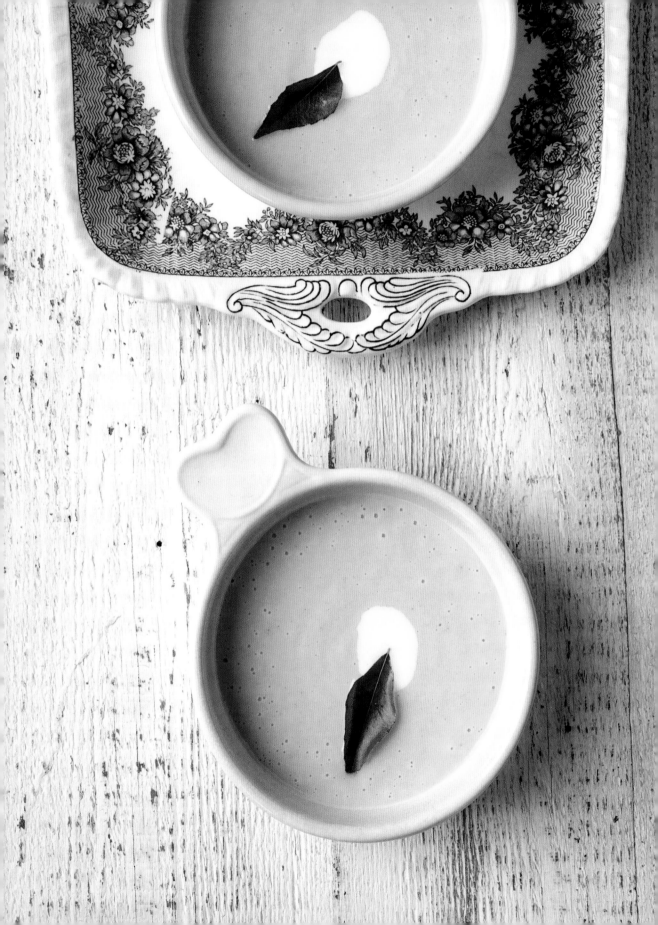

CHILLY SPICED APPLE

SERVES 4

1 tbsp olive oil

½ onion, sliced

600g Braeburn apples (or give
   whatever is in season a go)

½ tsp curry powder

500ml hot chicken or
   vegetable stock (pages 14–15)

juice of ½ lemon

100ml half-fat crème fraîche

4 curry leaves

flaky sea salt

This is the perfect soup for a sunny autumn weekend, when apples are plentiful and there is still warmth in the air after the morning mist has burned away.

Heat the olive oil in a large pan, add the onion and cook gently for 10 minutes or so, until softened. Meanwhile, peel, core and roughly chop the apples. After a few minutes, add the curry powder.

Once the onion is soft, add the hot stock and the apples. Bring to the boil, then reduce the heat to a simmer and cook for about 30 minutes, or until the apples are very soft. Season with salt and process in a blender until smooth. If you prefer a smoother soup, pass through a sieve before leaving it to cool.

Once cooled, add the lemon juice and crème fraîche. Taste to check the seasoning and serve at room temperature, or chilled if you prefer, garnished with curry leaves.

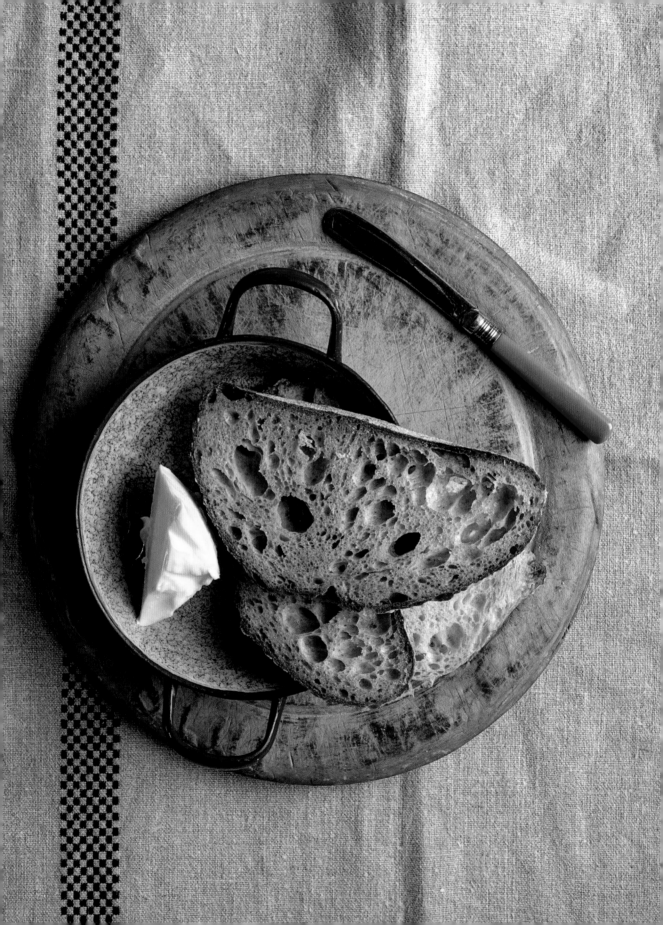

ON THE SIDE

Life without bread would be pale and uninteresting

If there's one thing we love too much, it's probably bread. Life without bread would be pale and uninteresting, and we try to add as much variety as possible in the flours we use when baking at home. For home baking, the So-Easy Soda Bread is incredibly fast and simple and yields warm, delicious loaves for the weekend. Likewise, Spelt Flatbreads are super-quick to knock up and can easily be made with any number of gluten-free flours for extra healthiness. Kate couldn't imagine how we were going to eat a bag of shelled hemp seeds that she bought in a fit of healthy-living enthusiasm, but she added them to oats and sesame seeds to make Sesame Seed and Hemp Oatcakes and surprised herself at how well they turned out.

The thing with any home baking is that when you eat bread or biscuits warm from the oven, they're going to taste amazing whatever you put in the mix. If you don't feel like baking, sourdough, which is available from most artisan bakers, is a good accompaniment to many of our soups, and is a little bit healthier than most breads because its wild fermented yeasts are more digestible.

SO-EASY SODA BREAD

MAKES 1 SMALL LOAF
(double up for family size
or to make 2 little loaves)

250g spelt or wholemeal flour,
    plus extra for dusting
1 tsp bicarbonate of soda
½ tsp flaky sea salt
200ml buttermilk
1 tablespoon natural yoghurt,
    if needed

If you've never baked bread before, start with soda bread and you'll never look back – it's just about the easiest thing in the world, and tastes amazing. Simple, plain spelt soda bread, as in this recipe, is lovely, or you could add pumpkin and sunflower seeds, walnuts, cranberries or a little honey.

Preheat the oven to 200°C/fan 180°C/400°F/gas mark 6.

Sift the flour and bicarbonate of soda into a large bowl and add the salt, giving it all a thorough mix. Make a well in the middle and gradually pour in the buttermilk, stirring constantly, to make a soft dough, that's just beyond sticky. Add some yoghurt if it looks a little dry.

On a lightly floured surface, knead the bread lightly for just a minute to make a loose ball. It doesn't need to be springy because there is no yeast to worry about. The main thing is to be quick so that the bicarbonate is still working when you put the bread in the oven (it is activated by liquid). Don't worry if there are cracks on top – these will make the bread lovely and crusty.

Put the dough on a floured baking tray and dust the top with more flour. Cut a deep cross in the top, then bake for 30 minutes, or until the loaf sounds hollow when tapped on the bottom.

Allow the bread to cool, as it will melt in the mouth after resting for a while. It's best eaten on the day you bake it, but if you wrap it in a tea towel it's very good toasted the next day – better than supermarket bread, for sure!

SPELT FLATBREADS

MAKES 4 FLATBREADS

125g white spelt flour, plus
    extra for dusting
a pinch of flaky sea salt
unsalted butter, to serve
    (optional)
sumac, to serve (optional)

These only take a minute to make, and don't contain any yeast. You can experiment with any unusual types of flour. Since they contain no preservatives, you need to eat them straightaway, but we don't mind that.

Put the flour in a large bowl and stir in the salt. Add 125ml water a little at a time, mixing and kneading all the time, until you have a soft, elastic dough. The more you knead it, the softer your flatbreads will be.

Turn the dough out on to a lightly floured surface. Divide the dough into 4 equal pieces and roll each one into a ball. Squash one ball down on the floured surface and roll it out to a thin disc about 15cm across. Repeat with the other pieces.

Heat a large frying pan and once it is very hot, place a flatbread on the pan and cook for 1 minute, or until it begins to bubble. Flip it over and cook the other side for about 30 seconds. Repeat for all 4 flatbreads. Serve immediately, with a little butter and sumac, if you like.

SESAME SEED & HEMP OATCAKES

MAKES ABOUT 20

100g medium oats
50g fine oatmeal
50g shelled hemp seeds
1 tbsp black or white sesame
   seeds
1/2 tsp flaky sea salt
50ml extra-virgin olive oil
flour, for dusting

Hemp seeds are a great source of protein and essential fatty acids, and contain the perfect balance of omegas 6 and 3, making these oatcakes the ideal companion to a vegetable soup.

Preheat the oven to 180°C/fan 160°C/350°F/gas mark 4 and line 2 baking trays with baking parchment.

Mix all the dry ingredients together in a large bowl. Make a well in the middle and pour in the olive oil, along with enough water to bring the ingredients together to form a dough. It should not be sticky, but bound together enough for you to be able to roll it out.

Turn the dough out on to a lightly floured surface and knead it lightly before rolling it out to about 5mm thick. Cut out rounds with a cookie cutter (8cm diameter is a good size) and arrange on the lined baking trays. Bake for about 30–35 minutes, or until crisp and golden. Remove from the oven and let stand for a few minutes, then transfer to a wire rack to cool.

RYE & CARAWAY BISCUITS

MAKES ABOUT 12

100g rye flour, plus extra for
    dusting
a large pinch of flaky sea salt
50g unsalted butter
1 tsp caraway seeds

We can both easily eat a whole packet of shop-bought crackers, but these homemade rye biscuits taste much richer, so you only need a couple with a hearty bowl of soup.

Preheat the oven to 180°C/fan 160°C/350°F/gas mark 4 and line a baking tray with baking parchment.

Mix the rye flour and salt in a large bowl, then rub in the butter with your fingertips until the mixture resembles breadcrumbs. Stir in the caraway seeds, then add enough water so that you can bring it together to form a dough – usually about 6 teaspoons. Turn the dough out on to a lightly floured surface and knead the dough gently.

Roll it out as thinly as you can and cut out round biscuits with a cookie cutter (8cm diameter is a good size). Place them on the lined baking tray, prick gently with a fork and bake for about 15 minutes, until dark golden. Remove from the oven and allow to cool for a few minutes before transferring to a wire rack to cool.

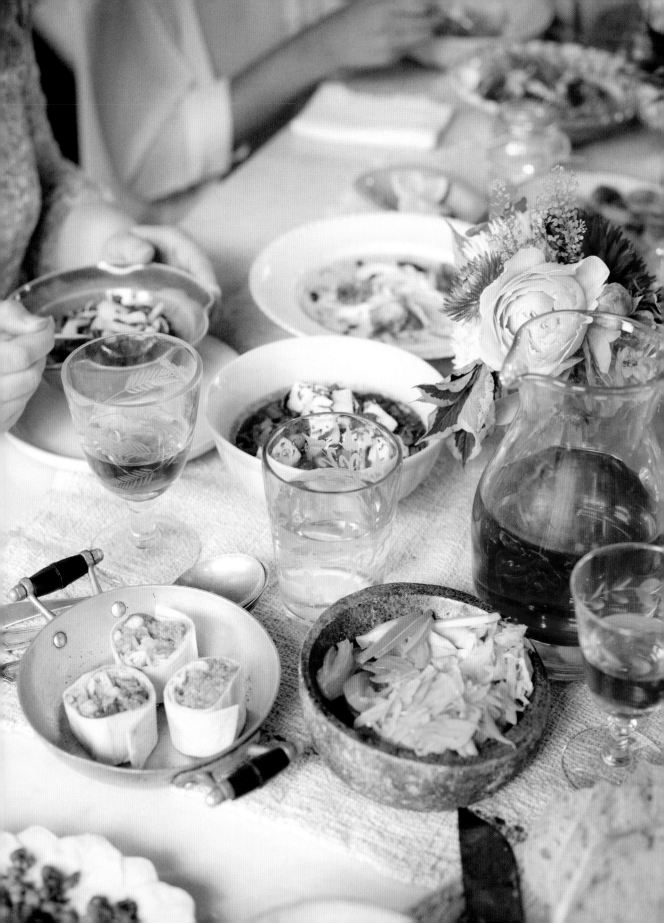

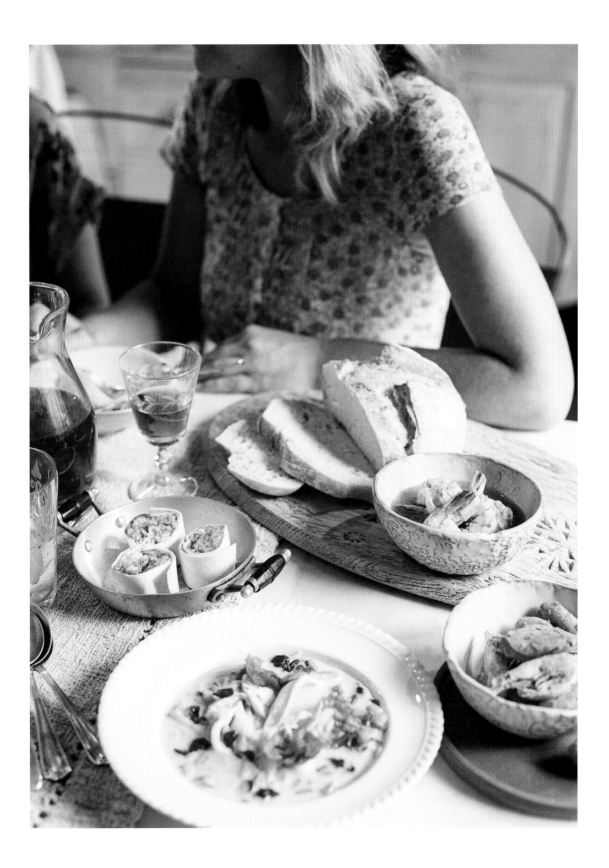

FAVOURITE RECIPE BOOKS & JOURNALS

We have rows and rows of cookbooks on our shelves at home, but these are the ones we reach for over and over again (except for *The Art of Fermentation* and *Salad*, both of which are recent additions, but which we're enjoying exploring). Michael Pollan is here because every time he writes a new book, we're reminded of the importance of food.

The Art of Fermentation by Sandor Ellix Katz (Chelsea Green Publishing, 2012)

The Art of Simple Food by Alice Waters (Michael Joseph, 2008)

Cereal magazine

Cooked: A Natural History of Transformation by Michael Pollan (Allen Lane, 2013)

Faviken by Magnus Nilsson (Phaidon Press, 2012)

Fields of Greens: New Vegetarian Recipes from the Celebrated Greens Restaurant by Annie Somerville (Bantam Doubleday Dell Publishing Group, 1998)

Instructions to the Cook: A Zen Master's Lessons in Living a Life That Matters by Bernie Glassman & Rick Fields (Shambhala Publications, 2013)

Kinfolk magazine

Salad by Yoshihiro Murata (Shibata Shoten, 2012)

Malouf: New Middle Eastern Food by Greg and Lucy Malouf (Hardie Grant Books, 2011)

The Modern Pantry by Anna Hansen (Ebury Press, 2011)

Plenty by Yotam Ottolenghi (Ebury Press, 2010)

Zenbu Zen by Jane Lawson (Murdoch Books, 2012)

RESOURCES

These are the online retailers we use for sourcing more unusual ingredients. We're also very lucky to live near a handful of health-food shops, organic grocers and Asian supermarkets, but if you don't, most things can be found online.

www.goodnessdirect.co.uk: A brilliant resource for grains, oils, beans and pulses if you can't get to a good health-food shop.

www.hookandson.co.uk: Find out all about raw milk straight from the farm.

www.japancentre.com: Perfect for stocking up on Asian ingredients, such as furikake, kombu, hojicha green tea and umebochi plums.

www.justingredients.co.uk: Supplier of teas, spices and Chinese herbs such as *dang gui* and *huang qi*.

www.martins-seafresh.co.uk: Incredible fish from Cornwall delivered to your door.

www.themodernsaladgrower.co.uk: Sean O'Neill has been growing organic salads for over 15 years, and now grows the most beautiful and delicious leaves and edible flowers.

www.natoora.co.uk: Quality fresh, seasonal produce, for when you need or fancy ingredients that are a bit special.

www.souschef.co.uk: For kimchi kits, Creole spice blend, sea spaghetti and much more.

www.thespicery.co.uk: An excellent-value range of individual spices and spice blends, and you can buy small pouches to avoid having jars of spices hanging around.

INDEX

ABOUT KATE & NICOLE

Kate and Nicole came together to create Food For Happiness (**www.foodforhappiness.co.uk**).

Kate Adams is a writer and founder of the Flat Tummy Club. She created the club after losing weight by finding the healthy things she loves (including soup), instead of trying to follow a strict diet regime. Five years later and Kate has kept the weight off and learned a lot about food, health and cooking along the way and as a result, the Flat Tummy Club is a thriving community. She was the health publisher at Penguin and now works with a number of experts across the health and wellbeing sectors.

Nicole Pisani is a chef who has worked at Yotam Ottolenghi's Soho restaurant NOPI and Anna Hansen's The Modern Pantry in London. Before that she ran a family restaurant in Malta, where people still stop her in the street to tell her how much they miss her rib-eye. When she was a baby, the first thing she picked up was an egg, and everyone knew she was going be a chef.

Coming together to write, cook and create, Kate and Nicole's aim is simply to help people become a little healthier and happier through the food they cook and eat. Food is at the foundation of creating good habits in our lives and cooking at home is a simple, unscientific, real-life answer to feeling happy about ourselves. Visit www.foodforhappiness.co.uk for recipes, events, cookery classes and more.

ACKNOWLEDGEMENTS

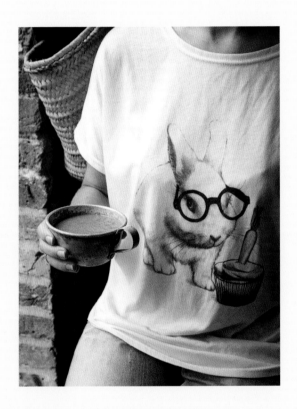

From Nicole
Thank you to the three important people who believed in me: Kate Adams, Thea Pisani, Cornelia Staeubli.

From Kate
Thank you Nicole for your creativity.

Thank you to the people involved in this beautiful book:
Kate Wanwimolruk, Amanda Harris, Clare Hulton, Regula Ysewijn, Tamzin Ferdinando, Helen Ewing, Caroline Clark and Laura Gladwin.

We make a good team.

First published in Great Britain in 2015
by Orion Publishing Group Ltd
Orion House, 5 Upper St Martin's Lane
London WC2H 9EA
An Hachette UK Company

10 9 8 7 6 5 4 3 2 1

A CIP catalogue record for this book is available from the British Library.

ISBN: 978-1-4091-5492-1

Design by Caroline Clark
Photography © Regula Ysewijn
Props by Tamzin Ferdinando
Copy-edit by Laura Gladwin
Project edit by Kate Wanwimolruk
Proofread by Jennifer Wheatley
Index by Hilary Bird

Printed and bound in Italy

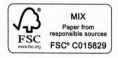

MIX
Paper from
responsible sources
FSC® C015829
FSC
www.fsc.org

www.orionbooks.co.uk

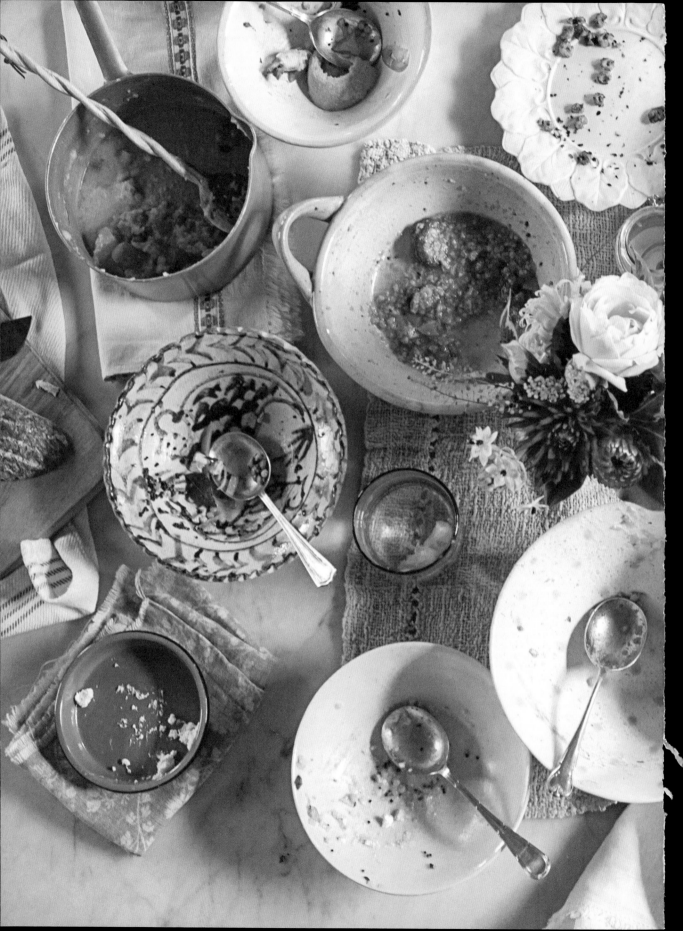